Contemporary Diagnosis and Management of

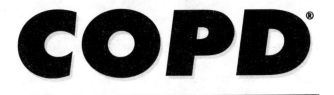

COPD®

Antonio Anzueto, MD

Professor of Medicine
University of Texas Health Science Center
and Director, Pulmonary Function Laboratory
Audie L. Murphy Memorial Veterans Hospital
San Antonio, Texas

Fernando J. Martinez, MD, MS

Professor of Medicine
and Director, Pulmonary Function Laboratory
University of Michigan Health System
Ann Arbor, Michigan

Published by Handbooks in Health Care Co.,
Newtown, Pennsylvania, USA

This book has been prepared and is presented as a service to the medical community. The information provided reflects the knowledge, experience, and personal opinions of the authors, Antonio Anzueto, MD, Professor of Medicine, University of Texas Health Science Center and Director, Pulmonary Function Laboratory, Audie L. Murphy Memorial Veterans Hospital, San Antonio, Texas, and Fernando J. Martinez, MD, MS, Professor of Medicine, and Director, Pulmonary Function Laboratory, University of Michigan Health System, Ann Arbor, Michigan.

International Standard Book Number: 1-931981-72-8

Library of Congress Catalog Card Number: 2006938240

Table of Contents

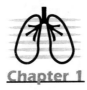

Chapter 1

Definition and Classification of Severity

The American Thoracic Society (ATS) and the European Respiratory Society (ERS) define chronic obstructive pulmonary disease (COPD) as "a preventable and treatable disease state characterized by airflow obstruction that is not fully reversible. The airflow limitation is usually progressive and is associated with an abnormal inflammatory response of the lungs to noxious particles or gases, primarily caused by cigarette smoking. Although COPD affects the lungs, it also produces significant systemic consequences."

A recent publication by the Global Initiative for Chronic Lung Disease (GOLD) recognized that COPD is a multicomponent disease characterized by chronic airflow limitation and a range of pathologic changes in the lung, some significant extrapulmonary effects, and important comorbidities that may contribute to the severity of the disease in individual patients. As a result, COPD should be regarded as a systemic disorder with significant comorbidities requiring a comprehensive diagnostic assessment of severity and appropriate treatment.

Chronic obstructive pulmonary disease is a complex disease that may have components of chronic bronchitis, emphysema, and asthma. Physicians caring for these patients have to be aware that recurring exacerbations are part of the natural history of this illness.

Chronic Bronchitis

Chronic bronchitis is defined clinically as chronic productive cough for 3 months in each of 2 successive years in a patient in whom other causes of productive chronic cough have been excluded. The increased production of sputum is a feature of this condition and is caused by goblet cell hyperplasia and airway inflammation.

Emphysema

Emphysema is defined pathologically as permanent enlargement of the airspaces distal to the terminal bronchioles, accompanied by destruction of their walls and without obvious fibrosis. In emphysema there is permanent destruction of the alveoli, the small elastic air sacs of the lung, because of irreversible destruction of a protein called elastin that is important for maintaining the strength of the alveolar walls. The loss of elastin also causes collapse or narrowing of the smallest bronchi, called bronchioles, which in turn limits airflow out of the lung.

Asthma and COPD

Asthma differs from COPD in its pathogenic and therapeutic response and should therefore be considered a different clinical entity. However, some patients with asthma develop poorly reversible airflow limitation. These patients are indistinguishable from patients with COPD and for practical purposes are treated as having asthma.

There is a high prevalence of comorbid asthma and COPD in the general population. This is characterized by significant airflow limitation and a strong response to bronchodilators. In these patients, the forced expiratory volume in 1 second (FEV_1) does not return to normal and frequently worsens over time. A great need exists to design studies aimed at determining the prevalence, natural history, clinical course, and therapeutic response in these patients.

Other Conditions

Poorly reversible airflow limitation associated with bronchiectasis, cystic fibrosis, and fibrosis caused by tuberculosis are not included in the definition of COPD and should be considered in its differential diagnosis.

Diagnosis Considerations

A diagnosis of COPD should be considered in any patient who has symptoms of cough, sputum production, or dyspnea, and/or a history of exposure to risk factors for the disease. The diagnosis requires spirometry; a postbronchodilator $FEV_1/$ forced vital capacity (FVC) <0.7 confirms the presence of airflow limitation. Spirometry should be obtained in all people with the following history: exposure to cigarettes, and/or environmental or occupational pollutants, and/or presence of the symptoms mentioned previously.

Because most COPD cases occur in patients who have smoked, all current or former smokers should be considered at increased risk for this disease. However, other risk factors, which account for fewer cases, include α_1-antitrypsin (AAT) deficiency, airway hyperresponsiveness, and indoor air pollution.

Patients with familial emphysema may have a hereditary deficiency of α_1-protease inhibitor. It is estimated that 1 in 3,000 newborns has a genetic deficiency of AAT, and 1% to 3% of all cases of emphysema are caused by AAT deficiency. The destruction of elastin that occurs in emphysema is thought to result from an imbalance between two proteins in the lung—an enzyme called elastase, which breaks down elastin, and AAT, which inhibits elastase. In a normal person, there is enough AAT to protect elastin so that abnormal elastin destruction does not occur. However, in a patient with inherited deficiency of AAT, the activity of the elastase is not inhibited and elastin degradation occurs unchecked. In those who smoke, 'smoker's emphysema' also results from an imbalance between elastin-degrading enzymes and their inhibitors. The elastase-AAT imbalance is thought to be a result of the effects of smoking, rather than an inherited deficiency. Studies of the effects of tobacco on the lung show that tobacco smoke stimulates excess release of elastase from cells normally found in the lung. The inhaled smoke also stimulates more elastin-producing cells to migrate to the lung, which in turn causes the release of more elastase. To make matters worse, free radical species and other oxidants found in cigarette smoke inhibit the elastase inhibitors and induce direct toxic effects. Therefore, there is a decrease in the amount of active antielastase available for protecting the lung, further upsetting the elastase-antielastase balance.

Classification of Severity

The GOLD and ATS/ERS recommend the classification of disease severity into four stages (Table 1-1). Patients with an $FEV_1/FVC > 0.7$ are considered at risk and should be encouraged to adopt a healthy lifestyle. Patients with a postbronchodilator $FEV_1/FVC < 0.7$ are considered to have COPD. The severity of the disease is then classified according to the predicted values obtained from validated population studies reflecting the individual patient demographic characteristics. The management of COPD is largely symptom driven, but the spirometric classification has proved useful in predicting health status, use of healthcare resources, development of exacerbations, and mortality. This classification is applicable to study populations and is not a substitute for clinical judgment in the evaluation of the severity of disease in individual patients.

Assessment of Severity

Although many patients are practically asymptomatic, persistent cough and sputum production often precede the development of airflow limitation. In some patients, the first symptom may be the development of dyspnea

Table 1-1: Spirometric Classification of COPD

Stage	Characteristics
Stage I: Mild COPD	FEV_1/FVC <70% FEV_1 >80% predicted With or without chronic symptoms
Stage II: Moderate COPD	FEV_1/FVC <70% 50%> FEV_1 <80% predicted With or without chronic symptoms
Stage III: Severe COPD	FEV_1/FVC <70% 30%> FEV_1 <50% predicted With or without chronic symptoms
Stage IV: Very Severe COPD	FEV_1/FVC <70% FEV_1 <30% predicted FEV_1 >50% predicted plus chronic respiratory failure

Modified from Celli BR, MacNee W, Agusti A, et al: Standard for the diagnosis and treatment of patients with COPD: a summary of the ATS/ERS position paper. *Eur Respir J* 2004;23:932-946. Global Strategy for the Diagnosis, Management, and Prevention of Chronic Obstructive Pulmonary Disease: GOLD Executive Summary. 2006 Update.

with previously tolerated activities. In the clinical course of the disease, systemic consequences such as weight loss, and peripheral muscle wasting and dysfunction may develop. Because of these and other factors, it is accepted that the single measurement of FEV_1 incompletely represents the complex clinical consequences of COPD. A staging system that could offer a composite picture of disease severity is highly desirable but is now not available. However, the variables listed in Table 1-1 have proved useful in predicting outcomes such as health status and mortality.

Suggested Readings

Celli BR, MacNee W, Agusti A, et al: Standard for the diagnosis and treatment of patients with COPD: a summary of the ATS/ERS position paper. *Eur Respir J* 2004;23:932-946. Available at: http://www.erj.ersjournals.com. Accessed November 7, 2006.

Connors AF Jr, Dawson NV, Thomas C, et al: Outcomes following acute exacerbations of severe chronic obstructive lung disease. The SUPPORT Investigators (Study to Understand Prognoses and Preferences for Outcome and Risks of Treatments). *Am J Respir Crit Care Med* 1996;15(4 pt 1):959-967.

Fabbri L, Pauwels RA, Hurd S, et al: Global Strategy for the Diagnosis, Management, and Prevention of Chronic Obstructive Pulmonary Disease: GOLD Executive Summary updated 2003. *COPD* 2004;1:105-141; discussion 103-104.

Feinleib M, Rosenberg HM, Collins JG, et al: Trends in COPD morbidity and mortality in the United States. *Am Rev Respir Dis* 1989;140 (3 pt 2):S9-S18.

Global Strategy for Diagnosis, Management, and Prevention of COPD. 2006 Update.

Higgins M. In: Cassaburi R, Petty TL. *Principles and Practice of Pulmonary Rehabilitation.* Philadelphia, PA, WB Saunders & Co, 1993, pp 10-17.

Higgins MW, Thom T. Incidence, prevalence and mortality: intra- and inter-country difference. In: Hensley MJ, Saunders NA, eds. *Clinical Epidemiology of Chronic Obstructive Pulmonary Disease.* New York, NY, Marcel Dekker, 1990, pp 23-43.

Higgins MW, Thom T. In: Hensley MJ, Saunders NA, eds. *Clinical Epidemiology of Chronic Pulmonary Disease*. New York, NY, Marcel, 1990, pp 22-43.

Mannino DM, Homa DM, Akinbami LJ, et al: Chronic obstructive pulmonary disease surveillance—United States, 1971-2000. *MMWR Surveill Summ* 2002;51:1-16.

Medicare and Medicaid statistical supplement, 1995. U.S. Department of Health and Human Services, Health Care Financing Administration. *Health Care Financ Rev Stat Suppl* 1995:1-388.

Pauwels RA, Buist AS, Calverley PM, et al: Global strategy for the diagnosis, management, and prevention of chronic obstructive pulmonary disease. NHLBI/WHO Global Initiative for Chronic Obstructive Lung Disease (GOLD) Workshop summary. *Am J Respir Crit Care Med* 2001;163:1256-1276.

Siafakas NM, Vermeire P, Pride NB, et al: Optimal assessment and management of chronic obstructive pulmonary disease (COPD). The European Respiratory Society Task Force. *Eur Respir J* 1995; 8:1398-1420.

Snow V, Lascher S, Mottur-Pilson C, et al: Evidence base for management of acute exacerbations of chronic obstructive pulmonary disease. *Ann Intern Med* 2001;134:595-599.

Standards for the diagnosis and care of patients with chronic obstructive pulmonary disease. American Thoracic Society. *Am J Respir Crit Care Med* 1995;152(5 pt 2):S77-S121.

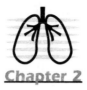

Epidemiology, Risk Factors, and Natural History

Chronic obstructive pulmonary disease (COPD) is a major public health problem. It is the fourth leading cause of morbidity and mortality in the United States and is projected to be the third leading cause of death worldwide in 2020 (Figures 2-1 and 2-2). The Global Initiative for Chronic Obstructive Lung Disease (GOLD) is a worldwide initiative to improve the knowledge of epidemiology, socioeconomics, public health, and health education of COPD.

The prevalence and morbidity of COPD greatly underestimate the total burden of the disease because it is usually not diagnosed until it is clinically apparent and moderately advanced (Figure 2-3). The worldwide prevalence of COPD in 1990 was estimated to be 9.34/1,000 in men and 7.33/1,000 in women. The number of people in the United States afflicted with COPD has risen sharply in recent decades. It is estimated that 4% to 6% of adult white males and 1% to 3% of adult white females have COPD. Estimates are that about 20 million patients have COPD, and that number has increased 41% since 1982.

Approximately 12.5 million people have chronic bronchitis. Among those with chronic bronchitis, the number who actually have airflow obstruction is unknown. In the United States in people 25 to 75 years of age, the estimated

1. Heart disease	724,269
2. Cancer	538,937
3. CVA	158,060
4. COPD	114,381
5. Accidents	94,828

Figure 2-1: Leading causes of death in the United States in 1998. NHLBI: *Morbidity and Mortality—2000 Chartbook on Cardiovascular and Lung Disease.*

prevalence of stage I, mild COPD was 6.9%, and of stage II, moderate COPD was 6.6%, according to the National Health and Nutrition Examination Survey (Figure 2-3). European data have similarly shown that 4% to 6% of the adult population have clinically relevant COPD. Studies from Germany, Spain, France, and Latin America have reported prevalence rates of 10% to 12%, 9.1%, 4.8%, and 7%, respectively (Figure 2-4). Thus, the number of patients with COPD may be underestimated because the condition is not widely recognized, and therefore may go untreated in a large number of the affected population (Figure 2-5).

The death rate from COPD in the United States has risen in recent decades in contrast with the falling death rates from heart and cerebrovascular diseases over the same interval (Figures 2-6 and 2-7). COPD is now the fourth most common cause of death in the United States, accounting for nearly 4.5% of all deaths in 1993, and has an estimated mortality of 100,000 patients. The data based on 1997 death rates attributable to COPD suggest that the areas with the highest death rates associated with COPD are the Northwestern states as well as New Mexico, Arizona,

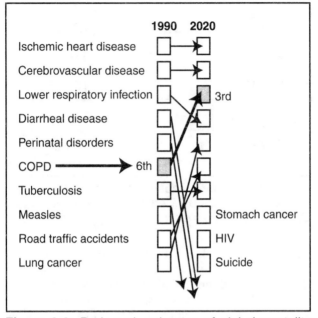

Figure 2-2: Projected estimates of global mortality in COPD, 2020. Modified from Murray CJ, Lopez AD: *Lancet* 1997;349:1436-1442.

and Nevada (Figure 2-8). These data may underestimate the mortality caused by COPD because death certificates commonly do not include COPD, despite reviews of medical records suggesting this diagnosis. Furthermore, COPD may be an important contributing factor in a large number of deaths, mainly people who die of coronary artery or cerebrovascular disease. The Centers for Disease Control and Prevention (CDC) recently reported the United States data regarding COPD mortality from 1980 to 2000. The data were obtained from the National Vital Statistics System. The most significant change during the period analyzed was the increase in COPD death rate for women, from

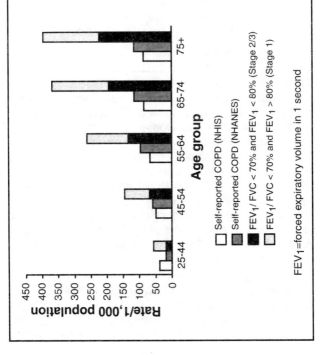

Figure 2-3: The estimated number and rates of people reporting COPD are presented above. The data show an appreciably greater prevalence of COPD in older vs younger individuals based on self-reporting. Additionally, data estimating the prevalence of COPD on the basis of spirometric definitions showed that for both mild and moderate COPD, the prevalence increased with age. Adapted from Manniano, *MMWR Surveillance Survey* 2002;51:1-16.

X axis: Age group — 25-44, 45-54, 55-64, 65-74, 75+

Y axis: Rate/1,000 population — 0, 50, 100, 150, 200, 250, 300, 350, 400, 450

Legend:
- Self-reported COPD (NHIS)
- Self-reported COPD (NHANES)
- FEV_1/ FVC < 70% and FEV_1 < 80% (Stage 2/3)
- FEV_1/ FVC < 70% and FEV_1 > 80% (Stage 1)

FEV_1=forced expiratory volume in 1 second

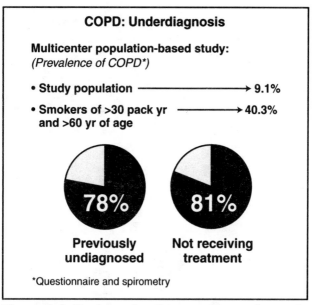

COPD: Underdiagnosis

Multicenter population-based study:
(Prevalence of COPD*)

- Study population ⟶ 9.1%
- Smokers of >30 pack yr ⟶ 40.3%
  and >60 yr of age

78%
Previously undiagnosed

81%
Not receiving treatment

*Questionnaire and spirometry

Figure 2-4: To determine the prevalence, diagnostic level, and treatment of COPD in Spain through a multicenter study comprising seven different geographic areas, 4,035 men and women (age range, 40 to 69 years) were randomly selected from a target population of 236,412 subjects. The prevalence of COPD was 9.1% (95% confidence interval [CI], 8.1 to 10.2%). The prevalence of COPD was 15% in smokers (95% CI, 12.8 to 17.1%); and 40.3% in patients who smoked more than 30 pack years and were older than 60 years. There was no previous diagnosis of COPD in 78.2% of cases (284 of 363), and 81% of all patients were not treated. Pena et al, *Chest* 2000;118:981-989.

20.1/100,000 in 1980 to 82.6/100,000 in 2000. In 2000, for the first time, the number of women dying from COPD surpassed the number of men dying from COPD (59,936 vs 59,118) (Figure 2-9). The death rates for COPD among

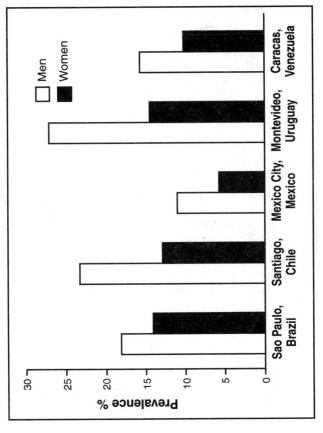

Figure 2-5: Prospective determination of the incidence of COPD in men and women in different cities of Latin America (PLATINO study). Menezes et al, *Lancet* 2005;366:1875-1881.

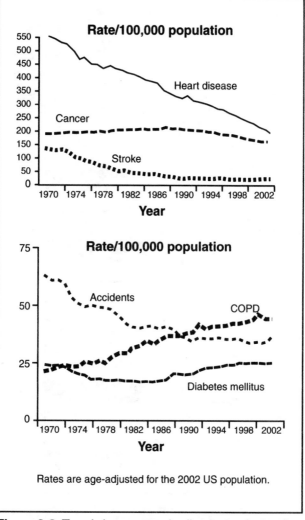

Figure 2-6: Trends in age-standardized rates for leading causes of death in the United States, 1970-2002. Jemal A: *JAMA* 2005;294:1255-1259.

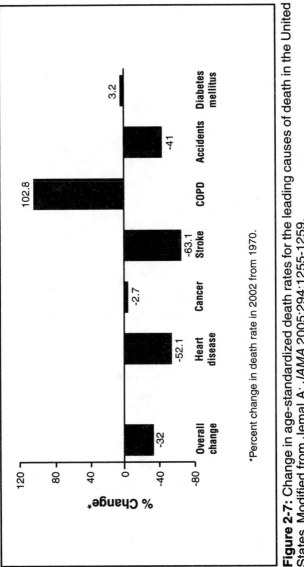

Figure 2-7: Change in age-standardized death rates for the leading causes of death in the United States. Modified from Jemal A: *JAMA* 2005;294:1255-1259.

*Percent change in death rate in 2002 from 1970.

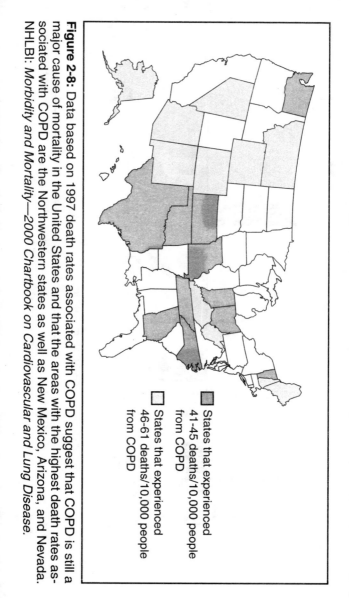

Figure 2-8: Data based on 1997 death rates associated with COPD suggest that COPD is still a major cause of mortality in the United States and that the areas with the highest death rates associated with COPD are the Northwestern states as well as New Mexico, Arizona, and Nevada. NHLBI: *Morbidity and Mortality—2000 Chartbook on Cardiovascular and Lung Disease.*

■ States that experienced 41-45 deaths/10,000 people from COPD

□ States that experienced 46-61 deaths/10,000 people from COPD

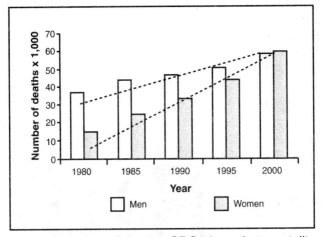

Figure 2-9: Data from the CDC show that mortality rates for COPD in women had a steep rise from 1980 to 2000. Manniano DM et al: *MMWR CDC Surveillance Summary* 2002;51:1-16.

men increased 13% from 1980 to 1985, but have remained steady since 1985. The incidence of COPD is known to vary between men and women and among ethnic groups—Caucasian, Hispanic, and African American. Of these groups, the highest mortality exists among white men and the lowest rates are among Hispanic women (Figure 2-10).

The economic and social burden of COPD is high. As a result of the morbidity of the disease, COPD expenditures for health costs were estimated at $37.2 billion in 2004, of which $20.9 billion were for direct costs. These direct costs for COPD included $8.6 billion for hospitalizations, $3.8 billion for physician services, $5 billion for prescription medications, and $2.8 billion for nursing home care (Figure 2-11). By comparison, the estimated total cost of asthma for 2002 was significantly less, at $14 billion, with $9.4 billion for direct cost. These costs have also been shown to vary based on patients' severity of disease. The most expensive

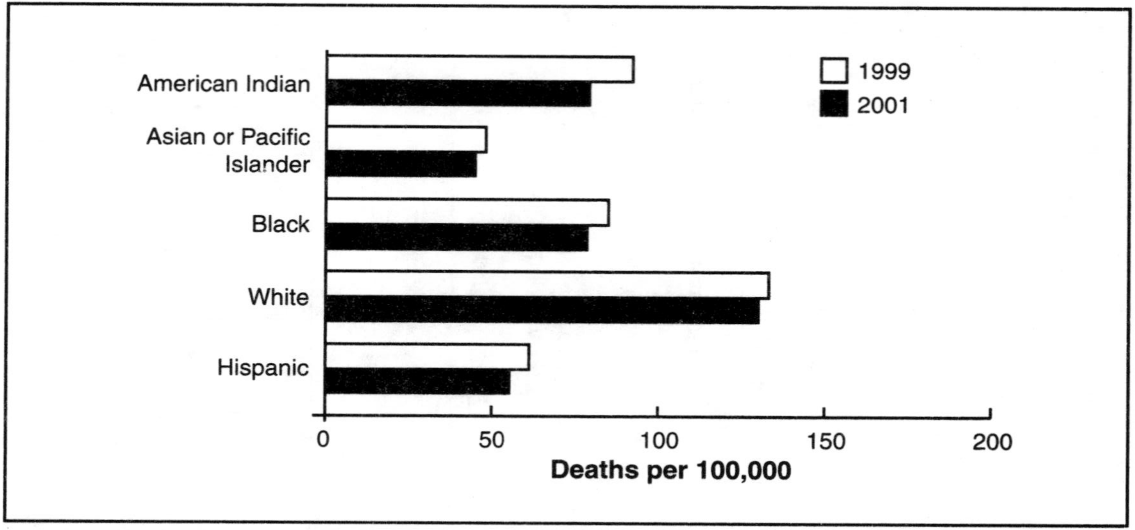

Figure 2-10: Data from the CDC show a slight trend in the reduction of death rate attributable to COPD in all race groups. However, it is noteworthy that the white population has the highest death rate attributable to chronic lower airway disease. Available at: http://www.cdc.gov.

22

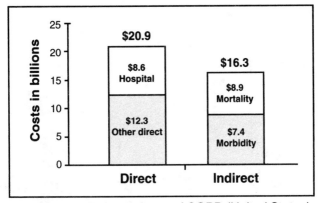

Figure 2-11: Estimated cost of COPD (United States), 2004. NHLBI: *Morbidity and Mortality—2004 Chartbook on Cardiovascular, Lung, and Blood Diseases.*

group are the patients with severe COPD, former ATS classification stage III (Figure 2-12). For a commercial insurer, health-care resource use among patients with COPD is at least double that of members of the same sex and age who do not have COPD. Recent studies using managed care administrative data demonstrated that COPD costs an average $420 to $657 per COPD patient per month, with acute hospitalizations comprising the largest proportion of these costs. Furthermore, this disease is also associated with significant disability. It is estimated that in 2020, COPD will be the fifth leading cause of disability-adjusted life years behind ischemic heart disease, major depression, traffic accidents, and cerebrovascular disease (Figure 2-13).

Risk Factors

The risk factors for developing COPD are active or passive cigarette smoking, family history of chronic lung disease, air pollution, occupational exposures, environmental allergic reactions, and recurrent respiratory infections, particularly during infancy (Table 2-1).

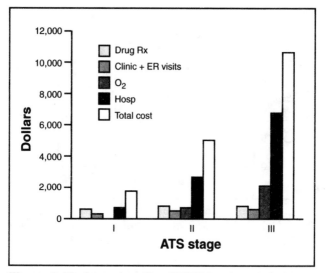

Figure 2-12: Annual median COPD treatment costs per patient, stratified by American Thoracic Society (ATS) severity stage. The data come from a retrospective pharmacoeconomic analysis of a cohort of 413 COPD patients. Hilleman DE et al: *Chest* 2000;118:1278-1285.

Smoking

Cigarette smoking is the main risk factor for COPD. The total number of active smokers has decreased by more than 50% in the adult population. This decrease has been particularly dramatic among white males. Approximately 50 million Americans continue to smoke, despite the fact that nearly half of all of the living adults in the United States who once smoked cigarettes have quit. Up to 3,000 people, mostly teenagers, start smoking daily. In fact, smoking is increasing among teenagers and young adults at a faster rate than in any other age group.

COPD is a progressive disease that results in decreased lung function and exercise capacity, and increased mor-

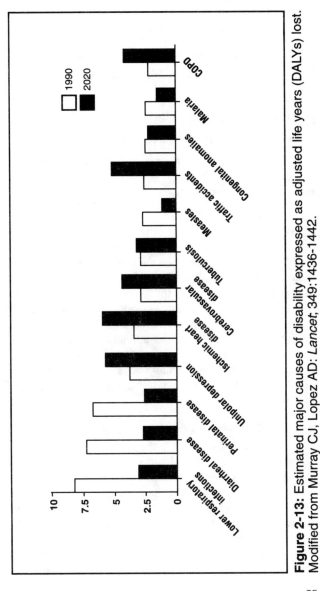

Figure 2-13: Estimated major causes of disability expressed as adjusted life years (DALYs) lost. Modified from Murray CJ, Lopez AD: *Lancet*; 349:1436-1442.

Table 2-1: Risk Factors for COPD

- Cigarette smoking—active and passive smoking
- Family history of chronic lung disease
- Air pollution
- Occupational exposures
- Environmental allergic reactions
- Recurrent respiratory infections, particularly during infancy

bidity, disability, and mortality (Figure 2-14). Smoking cessation has been shown to have major and immediate health benefits in altering the decline in lung function for men and women of all ages. Former smokers live longer than current smokers, and the benefits of quitting extend to those who quit at older ages. Smoking cessation at all ages reduces the risk of premature death. After 10 to 15 years of abstinence, the risk of all-cause mortality returns nearly to that of people who never smoked (Figure 2-15). In addition, many investigators have found in cross-sectional, population-based studies a lower prevalence of respiratory symptoms in former smokers compared with current smokers.

According to the 2000 National Health Interview Survey, 70% of adult smokers in the United States wanted to quit smoking. Predictors of success in smoking cessation include older age, male gender, higher income, lower levels of daily cigarette consumption, a history of past quit attempts, and a strong desire to stop smoking. In addition to the intrinsic characteristics of the smoker him/herself, smokers are more likely to successfully quit smoking when advised by a physician to stop. Several studies have demonstrated that former smokers have better health-

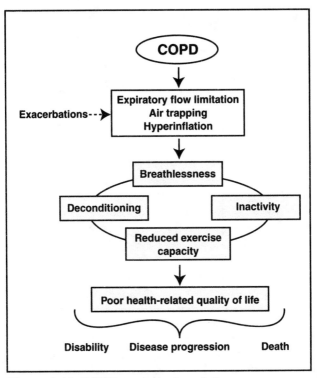

Figure 2-14: COPD: progression of disease.

related quality of life than current smokers as measured in a variety of ways, including days of illness, number of health complaints, and self-reported health status. In addition, former smokers, compared to current smokers, practice more health-promoting and disease-preventing behavior. Smoking is associated with an accelerated age-related decline in forced expiratory volume in 1 second (FEV_1), resulting in an annual loss of 80-100 cc per year compared with only 20 to 30 cc per year in a nonsmoker. Investigators have documented that smoking cessation

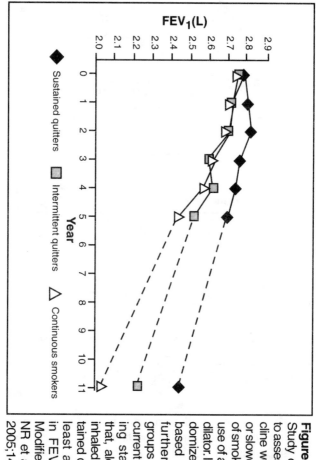

Figure 2-15: Lung Health Study of 5,887 individuals to assess whether FEV₁ decline would be halted and/or slowed through methods of smoking intervention and use of an inhaled bronchodilator. Individuals were randomized into three groups based on treatment, then further categorized into groups dependent on their current smoking/nonsmoking status. It was found that, along with use of an inhaled bronchodilator, sustained quitters showed the least amount of decline in FEV₁ over 11 years. Modified from Anthonisen NR et al: *Ann Intern Med* 2005;142:233-239.

is the only intervention to date that has proven to reduce this rate of decline in lung function (FEV_1) (Figure 2-15). In fact, with sustained abstinence from smoking, the rate of decline in lung function of former smokers returns to that of people who have never smoked. In addition, with sustained abstinence, COPD mortality rates and the mortality related to conditions such as coronary artery disease, lung cancer, and other medical conditions among former smokers decline in comparison with those who continue smoking (Figure 2-16).

The Vicious Cycle Hypothesis of Lung Destruction

Several authors have proposed a vicious cycle hypothesis to explain the clinical course of COPD. An infection (viral or bacterial) or a destructive agent such as an airborne pollutant is the usual trigger of the cycle (Figure 2-17). This initial event causes bronchial inflammation, which, in turn, damages the mucosal lining and impairs mucosal defenses, setting the stage for the next bacterial infection. This infection then intensifies the inflammation and results in further destruction of the mucosal wall, ultimately creating a larger surface area for bacterial growth and wall destruction. The inflammation causes bronchial wall edema, airway remodeling, bronchospasm, and mucus plugging. Because of weakened bronchial defenses, each exacerbation sets the stage for the next.

Acute exacerbations of COPD are associated with an additional increase in the airway inflammation burden (measured in sputum), especially in exacerbations associated with bacterial infections. There is a growing body of evidence that supports the vicious cycle hypothesis, showing that airway damage occurs when chronic infection or colonization with bacteria causes the host to continuously release inflammatory mediators. The host-response to infection is to release inflammatory cells found in sputum both in stable COPD and during exacerbations. These

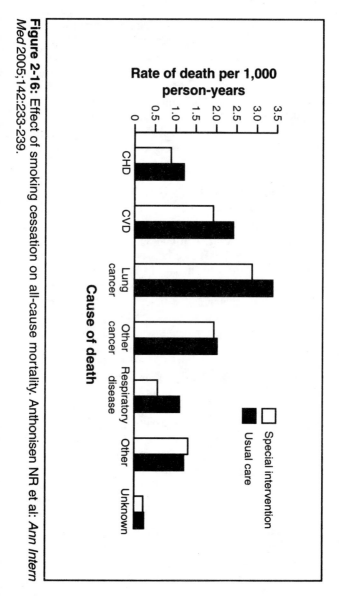

Figure 2-16: Effect of smoking cessation on all-cause mortality. Anthonisen NR et al: *Ann Intern Med* 2005;142:233-239.

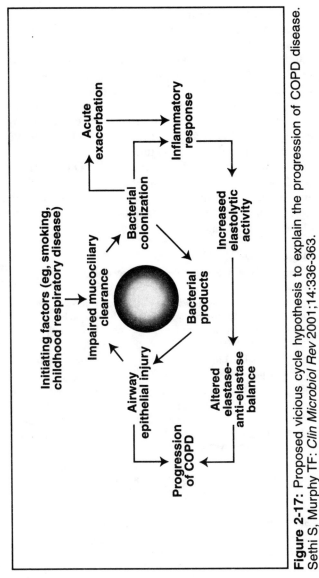

Figure 2-17: Proposed vicious cycle hypothesis to explain the progression of COPD disease. Sethi S, Murphy TF: *Clin Microbiol Rev* 2001;14:336-363.

cells are primarily neutrophils and macrophages. Inflammatory mediators that are significant in attracting these inflammatory cells to the airway are interleukin-6 (IL-6), interleukin-8 (IL-8), tumor necrosis factor-α (TNF-α), and leukotriene B_4 (LTB$_4$). End products of these inflammatory cells that mediate airway damage are neutrophil elastase (NE) and myeloperoxidase (MPO). Sputum inflammatory markers increase substantially during acute exacerbations of COPD and therefore could represent useful objective indicators of response to treatment. Recent observations have shown that the inflammation in COPD extends beyond the lung and that increased inflammatory markers are measurable in the serum, and further increase with exacerbations. Further understanding of the potential role of these markers in clinical care is needed.

Suggested Readings

American Thoracic Society: Pulmonary rehabilitation-1999. *Am J Respir Crit Care Med* 1999;15(5 pt 1):1666-1682.

Anthonisen NR, Connett JE, Kiley JP, et al: Effects of smoking intervention and the use of an inhaled anticholinergic bronchodilator on the rate of decline of FEV1. The Lung Health Study. *JAMA* 1994;272:1497-1505.

Ball P, Harris JM, Lowson D, et al: Acute infective exacerbations of chronic bronchitis. *QJM* 1995;88:61-68.

Bock BC, Goldstein MG, Marcus BH: Depression following smoking cessation in women. *J Subst Abuse* 1996;8:137-144.

CDC: Cigarette smoking among adults—United States, 2000. *MMWR* 2002;51:642-645. Available at: http://www.cdc.gov. Accessed November 14, 2006.

Celli BR, MacNee W, ATS/ERS Task Force: Standards for the diagnosis and treatment of patients with COPD: a summary of the ATS/ERS position paper. *Eur Respir J* 2004;23:932-946.

Covey LS, Glassman AH, Stetner F: Depression and depressive symptoms in smoking cessation. *Compr Psychiatry* 1990;31:350-354.

Duncan CL, Cummings SR, Hudes ES, et al: Quitting smoking: reasons for quitting and predictors of cessation among medical patients. *J Gen Intern Med* 1992;7:398-404.

Global Strategy for Diagnosis, Management, and Prevention of COPD. 2006 Update.

Fletcher C, Peto R: The natural history of chronic airflow obstruction. *Br Med J* 1977;1:1645-1648.

Freund KM, D'Agostino RB, Belanger AJ, et al: Predictors of smoking cessation: the Framingham Study. *Am J Epidemiol* 1992;135:957-964.

Hymowitz N, Cummings KM, Hyland A, et al: Predictors of smoking cessation in a cohort of adult smokers followed for five years. *Tob Control* 1997;6(suppl 2):S57-S62.

Mino Y, Shigemi J, Otsu T, et al: Does smoking cessation improve mental health? *Psychiatry Clin Neurosci* 2000;54:169-172.

Monso E, Campbell J, Tonnesen P, et al: Sociodemographic predictors of success in smoking intervention. *Tob Control* 2001;10:165-169.

Murphy SL: Deaths: final data for 1998. *Natl Vital Stat Rep* 2000;48:1-105.

Murphy TF, Sethi S: Bacterial infection in chronic obstructive pulmonary disease. *Am Rev Respir Dis* 1992;146:1067-1083.

National Institutes of Health. National Heart, Lung, and Blood Institute: Morbidity and mortality: 2002 chart book on cardiovascular, lung and blood diseases. National Heart, Lung, and Blood Institute. 2002 May 1 [cited: 2002 Sept. 19]. Available at: http://www.nhlbi.nih.gov/resources/docs/02_chtbk.pdf. Accessed November 14, 2006.

Pauwels RA, Buist AS, Calverley PM, et al: Global strategy for the diagnosis, management, and prevention of chronic obstructive pulmonary disease. NHLBI/WHO Global Initiative for Chronic Obstructive Lung Disease (GOLD) Workshop summary. *Am J Respir Crit Care Med* 2001;163:1256-1276.

Senore C, Battista RN, Shapiro SH, et al: Predictors of smoking cessation following physicians' counseling. *Prev Med* 1998;27:412-421.

Tillmann M, Silcock J: A comparison of smokers' and ex-smokers' health-related quality of life. *J Public Health Med* 1997;19:268-273.

United States. Public Health Service, Office of the Surgeon General, Office on Smoking and Health: The health benefits of smoking cessation: a report of the Surgeon General 1990. Issued by the performing agencies: U.S. Dept. of Health and Human Services, Centers for Disease Control, Center for Chronic Disease Prevention and Health Promotion, Office on Smoking and Health. DHHS Publication No: (CDC) 90-8416. Rockville (MD): U.S. Dept. of Health and Human Services.1999 [cited: 2003 Mar. 17]. Available at: http://sgreports.nlm.nih.gov/NN/B/B/C/T/. Accessed November 14, 2006.

Ware JE Jr, Kosinski M, Keller SD. *SF-36 Physical and Mental Health Summary Scales: A User's Manual.* Boston, MA, The Health Institute, New England Medical Center, 1994.

Wilson D, Parsons J, Wakefield M: The health-related quality-of-life of never smokers, ex-smokers, and light, moderate, and heavy smokers. *Prev Med* 1999;29:139-144.

Chapter 3

Pathology and Pathophysiology

hronic obstructive pulmonary disease (COPD) represents a syndrome complex characterized by the physiologic aberration of expiratory airflow limitation. As stated in international guidelines, this airflow limitation is "...not fully reversible, is usually progressive, and is associated with an abnormal inflammatory response of the lungs to noxious particles or gases, primarily caused by cigarette smoking." It is evident from this definition that an aggravated inflammatory response is considered a key biologic process in COPD.

Pathology

The pathologic processes underlying COPD have been described for decades, although the nature of these abnormalities has become clearer during the past several years. Evidence suggests that the host response to noxious stimuli (particularly cigarette smoke) generates a stereotypic response in susceptible patients. The resulting abnormalities involve the airways, alveoli, and pulmonary vessels within the lung. Figure 3-1 illustrates the changes seen within the smaller airways and the pulmonary parenchyma.

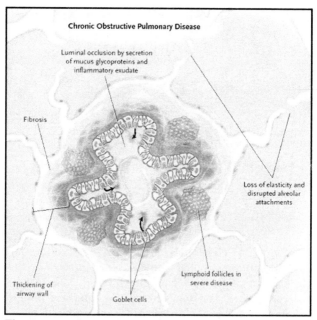

Figure 3-1: Response to noxious stimuli (eg, cigarette smoke) in the small airways and parenchyma of the lungs. Barnes PJ: Small airways in COPD. *N Engl J Med* 2005; 350:2635-2637.

Airway Changes

Chronic bronchitis is characterized by an inflammatory process that is located in the epithelium of the larger airways (>4 mm in internal diameter) and extends along gland ducts into the mucus-producing glands. The resulting abnormality is associated with increased mucus production, defective mucociliary clearance, disruption of the epithelial barrier, and thickening of the bronchial walls. Figure 3-2 (top panel) illustrates the enlarged glands typical of a patient with chronic bronchitis and the inflammatory infiltration of these glands (bottom panel; arrow and arrowhead). These changes are

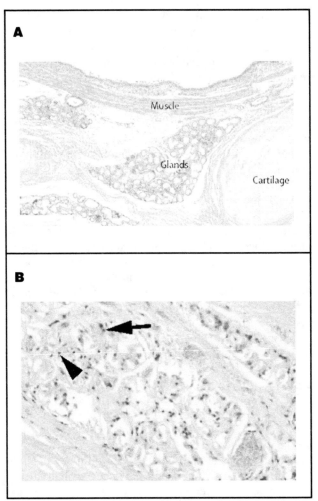

Figure 3-2: Panel A: Enlarged mucus-producing glands of a patient with chronic bronchitis. Panel B: Inflammatory infiltration of mucus-producing glands caused by chronic bronchitis. Hogg JC: Pathophysiology of airflow limitation in COPD. *Lancet* 2004;364:709-721.

associated with the typical symptoms of chronic bronchitis, including cough and sputum production occurring for at least 3 months during each of 2 consecutive years.

The clinical implications of such mucus hypersecretion remain controversial. Although some investigators have suggested that mucus hypersecretion is associated with a more rapid rate of fall in airflow, others strongly disagree. However, it is likely that hypersecretion is associated with greater use of health-care resources and, potentially, greater mortality. Chronic colonization and infection are commonly seen in COPD patients, particularly those with chronic mucus secretion. In fact, this mucus hypersecretion and chronic airway infection have been widely labeled 'The British Hypothesis,' which implicates these chronic findings as causative of the longitudinal deterioration in airway function in COPD patients. Such a process remains controversial but is the subject of intense investigation.

The importance of the smaller airways (<2 mm internal diameter) has been recognized for several decades since they were found to account for 10% to 15% of the total resistance to airflow in the normal canine lung. Similar data were subsequently reported in the human lung. More importantly, groundbreaking studies have confirmed that these airways are the predominant reason for airflow obstruction in COPD patients. Recent, innovative studies have expanded this concept. One investigative group analyzed lung tissue resected at the time of lung volume reduction surgery (LVRS) in patients with severe COPD. Tissue was collected remote from a lung-nodule resection in normal subjects and patients with mild-to-moderate COPD. Figure 3-3 (top panel) illustrates a small airway that is extensively remodeled by connective tissue in the subepithelial and adventitial compartments. Figure 3-3 (bottom panel) illustrates a direct relationship between worsening airflow obstruction (forced expiratory volume in 1 second [FEV_1]) and an increase in the thickness of the airway (expressed as the ratio of volume [V] and surface

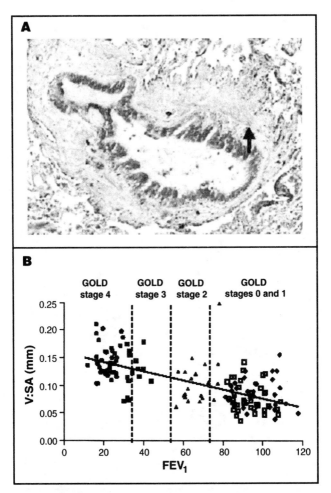

Figure 3-3: Panel A: Small airway extensively remodeled by connective tissue in the subepithelial and adventitial compartments. Panel B: Direct relationship between worsening airflow obstruction and thickness of airway. Hogg JC, Chu F, Utokaparch S, et al:The nature of small-airway obstruction in COPD. *N Engl J Med* 2004;350:2645-2653.

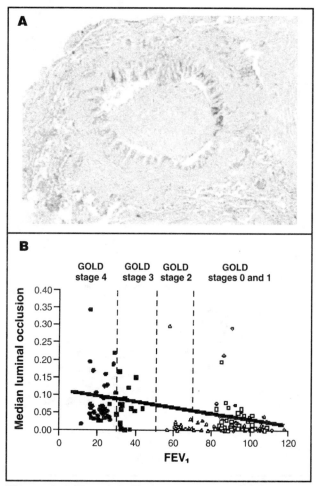

Figure 3-4: Panel A: Typical smaller airway with extensive luminal occlusion and airway resistance. Panel B: Relationship between increased luminal occlusion and increased airway resistance. Hogg JC, Chu F, Utokaparch S, et al: The nature of small-airway obstruction in COPD. *N Engl J Med* 2004;350:2645-2653.

area [SA]). These investigators also quantified the amount of luminal occlusion with mucus exudate. Figure 3-4 (top panel) illustrates a typical smaller airway with extensive luminal occlusion with mucus; the bottom panel illustrates the relationship between increasing luminal occlusion and increasing airway resistance (represented by lower FEV_1). These data provide a clear histologic correlate supporting the importance of small airway pathology in increasing airflow resistance in COPD.

Parenchymal Changes

Emphysema reflects an additional aberrant host response to noxious stimuli, most commonly cigarette smoke in developed countries. This destructive process is defined as "dilation and destruction of lung tissue beyond the terminal bronchiole." The type most commonly identified in smokers is centrilobular emphysema (see Figure 3-5, upper-panel diagram, high-resolution computed tomography [CT] image and histologic section). This abnormality is most commonly found in the upper lobes of the lung. Panacinar emphysema is usually associated with α_1-antitrypsin (AAT) deficiency and is generally more prominent in the lower lobes (Figure 3-5, lower-panel diagram, high-resolution CT and histologic image). There is a rough dose-response curve relating smoking exposure as enumerated by pack years of smoking and emphysema, although only about 40% of heavy smokers develop significant lung destruction. Substantial amounts of emphysema can be present in patients with normal lung function.

Systemic Changes

It has become increasingly evident that COPD is associated with a multitude of extrapulmonary manifestations. These include nutritional abnormalities and weight loss, skeletal muscle dysfunction, and cardiovascular effects, among others. Nutritional abnormalities have been described for many years and include alterations in caloric

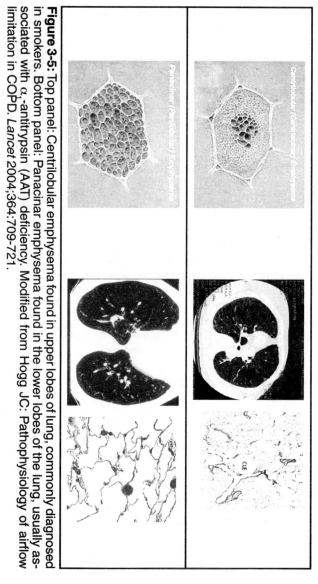

Figure 3-5: Top panel: Centrilobular emphysema found in upper lobes of lung, commonly diagnosed in smokers. Bottom panel: Panacinar emphysema found in the lower lobes of the lung, usually associated with α_1-antitrypsin (AAT) deficiency. Modified from Hogg JC: Pathophysiology of airflow limitation in COPD. *Lancet* 2004;364:709-721.

intake, basal metabolic rate, intermediate metabolism, and body composition. The most evident clinical manifestation of these changes is loss of skeletal muscle mass and unexplained weight loss. These features have proven to be powerful predictors of a worse prognosis for COPD patients. The skeletal muscle dysfunction is characterized by changes in fiber type composition and atrophy as well as decreased strength, endurance, and enzymatic activity. The abnormal muscle structure and function involve both the respiratory muscles and the peripheral muscles and are associated with impaired exercise capacity and quality of life.

Cardiovascular alterations are likely underestimated but important. These include impaired right-ventricular function in more severe disease, which is likely associated with a particularly poor prognosis. It has become increasingly evident that cardiovascular comorbidity, including ischemic disease, is important in COPD, such that even patients with milder COPD experience increased cardiovascular mortality. The nature of these systemic effects remains controversial and is under intense investigation. It is likely that a systemic inflammatory response is important (see next section). Increased circulating levels of inflammatory cytokines and acute-phase reactants, including interleukin (IL)-6, IL-8, tumor necrosis factor-α (TNF-α), and C-reactive protein (CRP), among others, have been reported by many groups. The increased CRP is particularly interesting, for a relationship between this elevated protein and ischemic cardiovascular disease has been widely reported.

Inflammation

The literature supporting an aggravated inflammatory response as a key biologic event in the COPD patient has burgeoned over the past decade. Numerous studies have confirmed the important role of inflammation in the airways and lung parenchyma in COPD. As COPD progresses, activated macrophages, neutrophils, and lymphocytes infiltrate

43

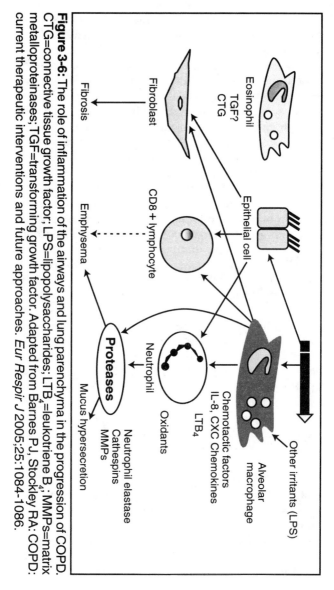

Figure 3-6: The role of inflammation of the airways and lung parenchyma in the progression of COPD. CTG=connective tissue growth factor; LPS=lipopolysaccharides; LTB$_4$=leukotriene B$_4$; MMPs=matrix metalloproteinases; TGF=transforming growth factor. Adapted from Barnes PJ, Stockley RA: COPD: current therapeutic interventions and future approaches. *Eur Respir J* 2005;25:1084-1086.

Eosinophil
TGF?
CTG

Fibroblast

Fibrosis

Epithelial cell

Emphysema

CD8 + lymphocyte

Other irritants (LPS)

Chemotactic factors
IL-8, CXC Chemokines

LTB$_4$

Alveolar
macrophage

Proteases

Neutrophil

Oxidants

Neutrophil elastase
Cathespins
MMPs

Mucus hypersecretion

44

the lungs (Figure 3-6). In contrast to asthma, eosinophils do not appear to be prominent participants in the inflammatory process in stable COPD patients. Eosinophils have been reported by some groups to be increased and activated during acute exacerbations.

Macrophages are key participants in the innate immune system, secreting cytokines and chemokines when stimulated by pathogen-associated molecular patterns (PAMPs). Many of the lung lymphocytes are type 1 cytokine-producing CD8+ T cells. These CD8+ T cells have been most evident in studies that used chronic bronchitis as the entry criterion, and are less evident when the study design selected against chronic bronchitis. Macrophages and lymphocytes are not only increased in the airways and alveoli of COPD patients, but the prevalence of these two cell types also correlates with the severity of airflow obstruction. Figure 3-7 illustrates the proportion of smaller airways with inflammatory cells as a function of increasing airflow obstruction (higher Global Initiative for Chronic Obstructive Lung Disease [GOLD] stages). The left panel illustrates the importance of neutrophils and macrophages; the bottom panel confirms a similar process for T and B cells.

Recent data have linked cigarette smoking and impaired activity of histone deacetylase (HDAC), which could aggravate the inflammatory process. The preponderance of literature supports that this ongoing inflammatory process is probably associated with the structural abnormalities found in the airways and parenchyma typical of COPD. Future investigation will shed further light on how this inflammatory process is perpetuated when smoking is discontinued and how novel therapeutic interventions can modulate this host response.

Pathophysiology

As stated earlier, expiratory flow limitation and increased airway resistance manifested by airflow obstruction are requisites for the physiologic definition of COPD.

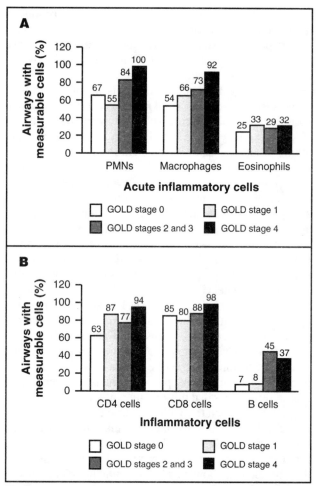

Figure 3-7: Inflammatory cells increase as a patient progresses through the GOLD stages. PMN=polymorphonuclear leukocyte. From Hogg JC, Chu F, Utokaparch S, et al: The nature of small-airway obstruction in chronic obstructive pulmonary disease. *N Engl J Med* 2004;350: 2645-2653.

The nature of this obstructive process is multifactorial and includes the luminal obstruction and fibrotic abnormality of the smaller airways, as well as emphysematous abnormality. The latter is associated with decreased elastic recoil and subsequent airflow obstruction. Expiratory flow limitation promotes hyperinflation, which can be particularly evident during exertion (dynamic hyperinflation). Figure 3-8 (panel A) shows that an increased end-expiratory lung volume (EELV) (reflected by the decreasing inspiratory capacity [IC]) is evident in a COPD patient compared with a normal subject.

This dynamic hyperinflation has been identified as an important determinant of exertional dyspnea in patients with COPD (Figure 3-8, panel B). A close relationship between increasing EELV (as a fraction of total lung capacity) and exertional dyspnea (as quantified by a Borg scale) is evident. Dynamic hyperinflation has been identified in COPD patients with mild airflow obstruction. The level of dynamic hyperinflation is related to the degree of workload and the minute ventilation (Figure 3-8, panel A). Patients with impaired gas exchange, who tend to exhibit a higher ventilatory response during exercise, experience increased dynamic hyperinflation and worse exertional dyspnea. Dynamic hyperinflation has numerous consequences, including increased work of breathing, functional impairment of the respiratory musculature, and adverse hemodynamic effects.

Conclusion

Chronic obstructive pulmonary disease reflects a syndrome of disorders unified by increased airway resistance. Airway resistance in turn reflects a series of structural abnormalities in the large and smaller airways as well as in the lung parenchyma. In addition, multiple systemic manifestations are evident and strongly influence health status and outcome. An aggravated and persistent inflammatory process is important to disease genesis, and probably to progression as well.

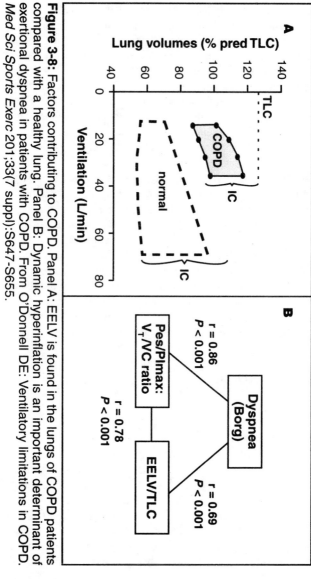

Figure 3-8: Factors contributing to COPD. Panel A: EELV is found in the lungs of COPD patients compared with a healthy lung. Panel B: Dynamic hyperinflation is an important determinant of exertional dyspnea in patients with COPD. From O'Donnell DE: Ventilatory limitations in COPD. *Med Sci Sports Exerc* 201;33(7 suppl):S647-S655.

Expiratory flow limitation promotes hyperinflation, which is particularly relevant during exertion. The resulting effect is exertional limitation with dyspnea. Therapeutic approaches now available effectively ameliorate dynamic hyperinflation. Future therapeutic agents will target the underlying biologic process, including the inflammatory process.

Suggested Readings

Agusti AG: COPD, a multicomponent disease: implications for management. *Respir Med* 2005;99:670-682.

Agusti AG: Systemic effects of chronic obstructive pulmonary disease. *Proc Am Thorac Soc* 2005;2:367-370.

Barnes PJ: Mediators of chronic obstructive pulmonary disease. *Pharmacol Rev* 2004;56:515-548.

Barnes PJ: Small airways in COPD. *N Engl J Med* 2004;350:2635-2637.

Barnes PJ, Cosio MG: Characterization of T lymphocytes in chronic obstructive pulmonary disease. *PLoS Med* 2004;1:e20.

Barnes PJ, Stockley RA: COPD: current therapeutic interventions and future approaches. *Eur Respir J* 2005;25:1084-1106.

Celli BR, MacNee W, ATS/ERS Task Force: Standards for the diagnosis and treatment of patients with COPD: a summary of the ATS/ERS position paper. *Eur Respir J* 2004;23:932-946.

Doherty DE: The pathophysiology of airway dysfunction. *Am J Med* 2004;117(suppl 12A):11S-23S.

Global Strategy for Diagnosis, Management, and Prevention of COPD. 2006 Update.

Hogg JC: Pathophysiology of airflow limitation in chronic obstructive pulmonary disease. *Lancet* 2004;364:709-721.

Hogg JC, Chu F, Utokaparch S, et al: The nature of small-airway obstruction in chronic obstructive pulmonary disease. *N Engl J Med* 2004;350:2645-2653.

Ito K, Ito M, Elliott WM, et al: Decreased histone deacetylase activity in chronic obstructive pulmonary disease. *N Engl J Med* 2005;352:1967-1976.

Martinez FJ, Standiford C, Gay SE: Is it asthma or COPD? The answer determines proper therapy for chronic airflow obstruction. *Postgrad Med* 2005;117:19-26.

O'Donnell DE: Ventilatory limitations in chronic obstructive pulmonary disease. *Med Sci Sports Exerc* 2001;33(7 suppl):S647-S655.

Shapiro SD: COPD unwound. *N Engl J Med* 2005;352:2016-2019.

Shapiro SD, Ingenito EP: The pathogenesis of chronic obstructive pulmonary disease: advances in the past 100 years. *Am J Respir Cell Mol Biol* 2005;32:367-372.

Vestbo J, Hogg JC: Convergence of the epidemiology and pathology of COPD. *Thorax* 2006;61:86-88.

Wouters EF: Local and systemic inflammation in chronic obstructive pulmonary disease. *Proc Am Thorac Soc* 2005;2:26-33.

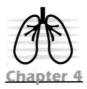

Chapter 4

Assessment of Disease

The diagnosis of chronic obstructive pulmonary disease (COPD) remains a clinical art, particularly because early diagnosis and appropriate staging are important. As noted in Chapter 1, the broad definition of COPD describes a syndrome of airflow obstruction that is not fully reversible in an individual with exposure to an identified risk factor. Chronic cough, sputum production, dyspnea, and chest tightness are the most common symptoms and so have diagnostic value. Cough is generally one of the first symptoms identified in COPD, while some investigators suggest that excess sputum production is associated with a decline in excess rate of forced expiratory volume in 1 second (FEV_1), an increased rate of subsequent hospitalization, and a greater impairment in quality of life. As such, patients with cough are appropriate candidates for early diagnostic testing to ensure an early diagnosis. Similarly, dyspnea is a frequent symptom that tends to negatively affect a patient's quality of life.

The physical examination can identify wheezing and prolonged expiratory phase but it is a crude and insensitive means of detecting more severe disease. In fact, a review of 44 studies assessing the value of clinical examination in diagnosing airflow obstruction identified no single item or combination of items that ruled out airflow obstruction. Although forced expiratory time can be helpful in suggesting the presence of disease, judging severity of disease by physical examination is notoriously difficult.

Physiologic Evaluation

Given the limitations of the clinical examination, it is evident that confirmation of airflow obstruction is required to ensure an accurate diagnosis. Fortunately, this is easily done with spirometry, a widely available, standardized, and relatively inexpensive diagnostic study. Spirometry is the most effective and reliable objective measure to confirm the diagnosis of COPD and is used to gauge disease severity (Table 4-1). It measures the maximal volume of air forcibly exhaled from the point of maximal inhalation (forced vital capacity [FVC]) and the FEV_1 of this maneuver. An individual's FEV_1 is considered to be in the normal range if it is at least 80% of the predicted value for that individual's age, sex, and height.

A COPD diagnosis can be made in patients with a postbronchodilator FEV_1 <80% of the predicted value in combination with an FEV_1/FVC <70%. Recently, the use of the FEV_6 has been advocated as a simpler, more reproducible marker than the FVC. Spirometric techniques have been standardized and widely available predicted equations are available for normal values. It is important that appropriate attention be given to good technique because some investigators have identified difficulties with the quality of spirometry in the primary care setting. When used appropriately, however, spirometric data significantly improve COPD detection in the primary care setting and alter decision making.

The presence and extent of bronchoreversibility and its diagnostic value in COPD remain controversial topics. In fact, some degree of bronchoreversibility is often seen in patients meeting diagnostic criteria for COPD. Interestingly, some have suggested that bronchoreversibility in COPD is associated with increased sputum eosinophilia, a picture

Table 4-1: Spirometric Classification of COPD

Stage	Characteristics
Stage I: Mild COPD	FEV_1/FVC <70% FEV_1 >80% predicted With or without chronic symptoms
Stage II: Moderate COPD	FEV_1/FVC <70% 50%> FEV_1 <80% predicted With or without chronic symptoms
Stage III: Severe COPD	FEV_1/FVC <70% 30%> FEV_1 <50% predicted With or without chronic symptoms
Stage IV: Very Severe COPD	FEV_1/FVC <70% FEV_1 <30% predicted FEV_1 >50% predicted plus chronic respiratory failure

Modified from Celli BR, et al: *Eur Respir J* 2004;23:932-946. Global Strategy for the Diagnosis, Management, and Prevention of Chronic Obstructive Pulmonary Disease: GOLD Executive Summary. 2006 Update.

more typical of asthma (see below). Complete bronchoreversibility argues against the diagnosis of COPD, although an inflammatory process in the pulmonary parenchyma or airways in response to a risk factor may still be present.

The measurement of diffusing capacity of the lung for carbon monoxide (DLCO) should be considered a routine test in the evaluation of chronic airflow obstruction, particularly in more advanced disease. The DLCO has been established as a sensitive test in the detection of emphysema, which is associated with loss of alveolar surface area and pulmonary circulation. The specificity of the test is low, however, and its use must complement a thorough clinical history and physical examination. Although not completely accurate in suggesting the presence of emphysema, a decreased DLCO in a patient with chronic airflow obstruction suggests a component of pathologic emphysema. As such, measurement of DLCO has diagnostic value in establishing an accurate diagnosis in patients with chronic airflow obstruction.

More recently, novel physiologic techniques have been used to characterize patients with COPD. Detailed assessment of flow limitation during tidal expiration has been shown to better correlate with symptoms and exercise limitation. Unfortunately, the technical requirements of this testing preclude its widespread use in clinical practice. Increasingly, the importance of dynamic change in operational lung volumes during exercise in COPD has been recognized. In contrast to normal subjects, during exercise COPD patients (particularly those with worse severity of airflow obstruction) exhibit a dynamic increase in lung volume at end expiration. The physiologic consequences of such a response include negative cardiovascular effects and impaired respiratory muscle function. In fact, the presence of exertional dyspnea closely correlates with this rise in exertional lung volumes. Although such testing has become increasingly available and used to define response to various therapeutic interventions in COPD, it is not now widely available in general practice. On the other hand, elevated static lung volumes correlate roughly with additional increase in lung volume during exertion. Furthermore, increased static lung volumes appear to be correlated with impaired prognosis in COPD. Therefore, clinicians may increasingly rely on routine measurement of lung volume in the future.

Radiologic Evaluation

Radiologic studies have assumed an increasing role in the evaluation of patients with COPD, particularly computed tomography (CT). This technique provides excellent visual, anatomic detail for detecting, characterizing, and quantitatively determining the severity of emphysema. High-resolution CT (HRCT) is more accurate than conventional CT. Furthermore, emphysema severity on HRCT correlates well with the pathologic severity of emphysema. Similarly, quantitative analysis of emphysema correlates with decreasing DLCO and is useful in identifying emphysema, usually mild, in patients with an isolated decrement in DLCO.

The clinical role of HRCT in the evaluation of COPD has best been established for the evaluation of surgical therapies. HRCT imaging has assumed a primary role in the evaluation of patients for lung volume reduction surgery (LVRS). The presence of heterogeneous, upper-lobe predominant emphysema as defined by HRCT has become widely accepted as the primary determinant of response to bilateral LVRS. Similarly, CT has become an integral part of the evaluation of COPD patients for lung transplantation. The presence of nodules and disease severity clearly alters decision making in this setting.

More recently, CT has been increasingly used to identify small airway abnormalities that correlate with those identified in histologic specimens (see Chapter 3). In this way, some investigative groups have divided patients with COPD into those with a predominantly emphysematous phenotype, those with predominant airway abnormalities, and those with mixed features. The clinical implications of such findings are unclear but it is likely that such imaging approaches will assume a greater clinical role in the future.

Differential Diagnosis

The role of diagnostic testing remains controversial in identifying features of asthma, emphysema, chronic bronchitis, or chronic bronchiolitis in individual patients. Although asthma is not considered in the diagnosis of COPD, in clinical practice these diseases are not discrete entities and demonstrate significant overlap (Table 4-2). Although there are unique features of the inflammatory process in well-defined asthmatics, significant overlap can be seen with COPD patients in clinical practice. One study retrospectively examined 547 consecutive adult patients, separating them into those with a primary diagnosis of asthma (n=337) or with COPD (n=210). Importantly, 20% of the population exhibited clinical and physiologic features of *both* disorders, confirming the clinical difficulty in segregating patients into distinct diagnostic categories.

A multivariate model to diagnose COPD suggested that the age at onset, male gender, smoking status, atopy status, and productive cough were the most useful clinical features. Similarly, a prospective study of adult patients with a history consistent with obstructive lung disease in numerous primary care practices confirmed that in those patients with spirometrically defined COPD most reported a previous diagnosis of asthma. A gender bias in diagnosing COPD has been supported by two studies of primary care clinicians; a typical clinical-physiologic picture of COPD was more likely to be diagnosed as asthma if the hypothetical case was presented as a female in contrast to a male.

These diagnostic difficulties have led to an increasing body of literature regarding the differential diagnostic approach to a patient with COPD (Table 4-2). As noted earlier, patients with a younger age at the onset of respiratory symptoms are more likely to have asthma. An exception to this is α_1-antitrypsin (AAT) deficiency, where significant emphysema can be seen at a young age. Similarly, the presence of atopy or variable symptoms supports a diagnosis of asthma. The role of spirometry in the differential diagnosis of asthma vs COPD was alluded to earlier. Complete reversal of airflow obstruction after bronchodilator administration or after a short course of steroid therapy argues against a COPD diagnosis. Less impressive reversibility creates diagnostic uncertainty because patients with COPD may demonstrate partial bronchoreversibility, while some patients with well-defined asthma exhibit incomplete bronchoreversibility. One evidence-based guideline has suggested that a rise in FEV_1 >400 cc after a bronchodilator suggests an underlying diagnosis of asthma.

The measurement of DLCO may provide additional information. In general, the DLCO is normal or elevated in asthma. Although not completely accurate in suggesting the presence of emphysema, a decreased DLCO in the setting of chronic airflow obstruction suggests a component of pathologic emphysema. As such, in large epidemiologic studies the presence of a normal DLCO has been associated with a clinical syndrome more consistent with asthma. On the other hand, DLCO measurement has potential limits in differentiating asthma from emphysema; for example, one group reported a DLCO lower than 80% predicted in four of 14 asthmatics with incompletely reversible airflow obstruction. Although HRCT can be used to assess the presence of emphysema or small airway abnormality, its clinical role in the routine diagnostic approach to COPD vs asthma remains unclear.

It is important to consider a focused diagnostic approach to patients with airflow obstruction because the therapeutic approach to asthma compared to COPD likely differs (Figure 4-1). Furthermore, there is likely a different rate of progression and mortality in patients with asthma vs COPD.

Monitoring

Because COPD is generally a progressive disorder, close serial monitoring is important in optimizing therapeutic interventions. Symptomatic monitoring includes

Table 4-2: Biologic and Clinical Features Contrasting Asthma With COPD

Feature	Asthma
Biologic	
Cellular infiltration	Eosinophils
	CD4+ lymphocytes
	Activated mast cells
Mediators	LTD_4
	IL-4, IL-5
Structural consequences	Fragile epithelium
	Thickened basement membrane
	Mucus metaplasia
	Glandular enlargement
Clinical	
	Early onset (<40 years)
	Varying or intermittent symptoms
	Nighttime symptoms
	Presence of atopy
	Family history
Physiologic	
	Airflow limitation that is largely reversible
	Airway hyper-responsiveness is significant

IL-4=interleukin-4
IL-5=interleukin-5 LTB_4=leukotriene B_4
IL-6=interleukin-6 LTD_4=leukotriene D_4

COPD

Neutrophils
Macrophages
CD8+ lymphocytes
CD4+ lymphocytes
Eosinophils

LTB_4
IL-8
TNF-α

Squamous metaplasia of epithelium
Parenchymal destruction
Mucus metaplasia
Glandular enlargement
Peribronchiolar fibrosis

Midlife onset
Slowly progressive symptoms
Prominent smoking history

Airflow limitation that is
 incompletely reversible
Airway hyperresponsiveness
 variable

Adapted from Martinez et al: *Postgrad Med* 2005;117:19-26.

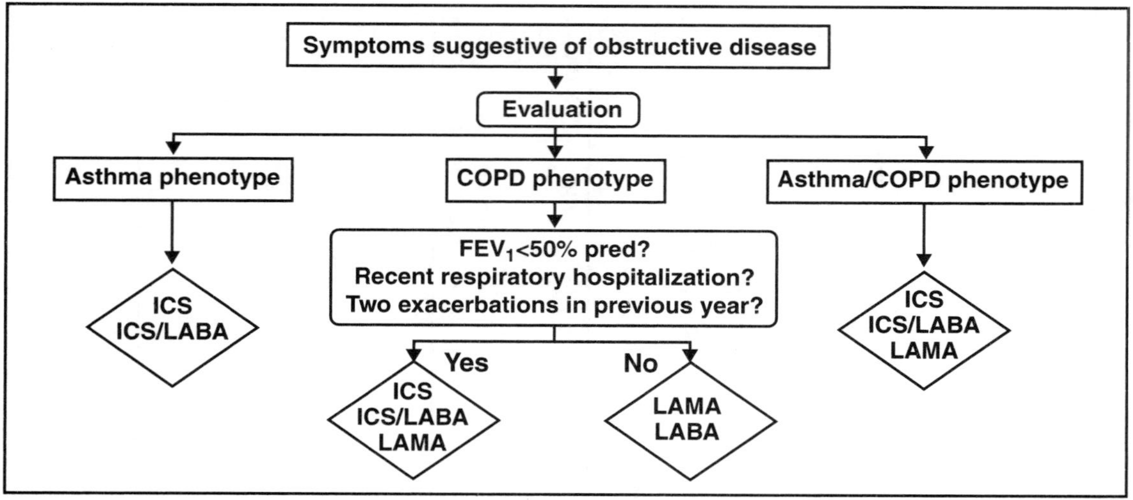

Figure 4-1: Potential algorithmic approach to a patient with symptoms suggestive of an obstructive disorder. COPD = chronic obstructive pulmonary disease; ICS = inhaled corticosteroid, LAMA = long-acting antimuscarinic agent, LABA = long-acting β-agonist. Modified from Martinez et al: *Postgrad Med* 2005;117:19-26.

quantifying the severity and frequency of cough and dyspnea. Similarly, identifying and treating exacerbations of disease are important interventions because these acute deteriorations in clinical status have a significant effect on pulmonary function, which can take several weeks to recover. Furthermore, exacerbations have a significant impact on impaired quality of life in these patients. The role of serial physiologic monitoring remains poorly defined, although serial spirometric monitoring may provide a diagnostic advantage over a single test. Furthermore, it is important to keep in mind that patients with COPD are at risk of developing other smoking-related illnesses such as bronchogenic carcinoma and coronary artery disease.

Suggested Readings

Beeh KM, Kornmann O, Beier J, et al: Clinical application of a simple questionnaire for the differentiation of asthma and chronic obstructive pulmonary disease. *Respir Med* 2004;98:591-597.

Buffels J, Degryse J, Heyrman J, et al: Office spirometry significantly improves early detection of COPD in general practice: the DIDASCO Study. *Chest* 2004;125:1394-1399.

Calverley PM, Koulouris NG: Flow limitation and dynamic hyperinflation: key concepts in modern respiratory physiology. *Eur Respir J* 2005;25:186-199.

Celli BR, MacNee W, ATS/ERS Task Force: Standards for the diagnosis and treatment of patients with COPD: a summary of the ATS/ERS position paper. *Eur Respir J* 2004;23:932-946.

Chapman KR, Tashkin DP, Pye DJ: Gender bias in the diagnosis of COPD. *Chest* 2001;119:1691-1695.

Cooper CB: Assessment of pulmonary function in COPD. *Sem Respir Crit Care Med* 2005;26:246-252.

Dales RE, Vandemheen KL, Clinch J, et al: Spirometry in the primary care setting: influence on clinical diagnosis and management of airflow obstruction. *Chest* 2005;128:2443-2447.

Eaton T, Withy S, Garrett JE, et al: Spirometry in primary care practice: the importance of quality assurance and the impact of spirometry workshops. *Chest* 1999;116:416-423.

Flaherty KR, Martinez FJ. The role of computed tomography in emphysema and lung volume reduction surgery. In: Lipson D, van Beek E, eds. *Functional Lung Imaging, Lung Biology in Health and Disease*. Boca Raton, FL, Taylor & Francis Group, 2005, pp 431-451.

Global Strategy for Diagnosis, Management, and Prevention of COPD. 2006 Update.

Holleman DR Jr, Simel DL: Does the clinical examination predict airflow limitation? *JAMA* 1995;273:313-319.

Kitaguchi Y, Fujimoto K, Kubo K, et al: Characteristics of COPD phenotypes classified according to the findings of HRCT. *Respir Med* 2006;100:1742-1752.

Kotloff RM, Lipson DA. Lung transplantation: radiographic considerations. In: Lipson D, van Beek E, eds. *Functional Lung Imaging. Lung Biology in Health and Disease*. Boca Raton, FL, Taylor & Francis Group, 2005, pp 593-620.

Martinez FJ, Standiford C, Gay SE: Is it asthma or COPD? The answer determines proper therapy for chronic airflow obstruction. *Postgrad Med* 2005;117:19-26.

Miller MR, Hankinson J, Brusasco V, et al: Standardisation of spirometry. *Eur Respir J* 2005;26:319-338.

Miravitlles M, de la Roza C, Naberan K, et al: Attitudes toward the diagnosis of chronic obstructive pulmonary disease in primary care. *Arch Bronconeumol* 2006;42:3-8.

National Collaborating Centre for Chronic Conditions: Chronic obstructive pulmonary disease. National clinical guideline on management of chronic obstructive pulmonary disease in adults in primary and secondary care. *Thorax* 2004;59(suppl 1):1-232.

Pellegrino R, Viegi G, Brusasco V, et al: Interpretative strategies for lung function tests. *Eur Respir J* 2005;26:948-968.

Schermer TR, Jacobs JE, Chavannes NH, et al: Validity of spirometric testing in a general practice population of patients with chronic obstructive pulmonary disease (COPD). *Thorax* 2003; 58:861-866.

Tinkelman DG, Price DB, Nordyke RJ, et al: Misdiagnosis of COPD and asthma in primary care patients 40 years of age and over. *J Asthma* 2006;43:75-80.

Chapter 5

Reducing Risk Factors

C hronic obstructive pulmonary disease (COPD) reflects a stereotypical response in the lung parenchyma and airways to an injurious agent. It is clear that host response to injury attenuates this response. Numerous injurious agents have been implicated in this response (Table 5-1). A comprehensive approach to COPD management requires an understanding of the role of risk factors in COPD genesis and how exposure to these risk factors can be modified.

Risk Factors for COPD
Cigarette Smoking
Much of the evidence addressing the role of cigarette smoking in COPD comes from cross-sectional studies, although several large longitudinal studies have shed important light. The most instructive of these is the Lung Health Study. This multicenter investigation randomized 5,887 smokers, 35 to 60 years of age, with spirometric evidence of mild airflow obstruction, to an intensive smoking intervention vs usual care. Over the initial 5-year follow-up period, subjects in the smoking cessation intervention groups exhibited significantly smaller declines in the forced expiratory volume in 1 second (FEV_1) than those in the control group. Eleven years after entry into the study, more than three quarters of the subjects underwent repeat spirometric testing; subjects who continued to smoke

Table 5-1: Exposures Implicated in the Development of COPD

- Tobacco smoke
- Occupational dusts
- Occupational chemicals
- Air pollution (indoor and outdoor)
- Infectious agents

exhibited a markedly higher yearly lung function decline than those who were in the usual care group. Interestingly, improvements in pulmonary function with smoking cessation were more evident among female subjects. Additional important results have been published from this groundbreaking longitudinal study. After 14.5 years of follow-up, all-cause mortality was significantly lower in the smoking cessation group, a difference that was particularly marked in sustained quitters; these differences were particularly evident among the heaviest smokers. The majority of deaths in the study related to cardiovascular causes and lung cancers. Amelioration of lung function loss was only seen in those subjects with dramatic reductions in smoking decrease (>85% reduction). The totality of these data supports the association of cigarette smoking with excess loss of lung function, increased respiratory symptoms, and increased mortality.

Importantly, not all smokers develop physiologic evidence of COPD. Although many have suggested that only about 15% of smokers appear to be at risk, recent analyses of available data suggest that this is an underestimate; some have suggested that the rate may be much closer to 50%. Although the topic remains controversial, numerous investigators have suggested that this risk is higher in female smokers. A genetic predisposition is likely.

Other Environmental and Occupational Exposures

Increasingly, it has been noted that a large minority of patients diagnosed with COPD have no smoking history. A recent multinational, Latin American study confirmed that the prevalence of COPD among nonsmokers ranged from 6.2% to 15.9%. An analysis of the Third National Health and Nutrition Examination Survey suggested that 23% of the total burden of airflow obstruction was seen in nonsmokers; 19% of these reported a prior diagnosis of asthma, 12.5% a prior diagnosis of COPD, while 68.5% reported no prior respiratory diagnosis. A separate analysis of the same database suggested that one quarter of mild and moderate-to-severe cases were nonsmokers. In fact, an ad hoc committee of the American Thoracic Society (ATS) reviewed population-based studies and suggested a population-attributable risk for occupational exposure in COPD of approximately 15% to 20%. The biologic nature of this airflow obstruction remains unclear but some may relate to environmental tobacco smoke exposure.

Occupational air dust exposure is the best known additional risk factor for COPD. Cross-sectional and longitudinal studies have implicated numerous causative agents (Table 5-2). In fact, some of these studies have suggested that the effect of occupational exposure is similar to that of moderate cigarette smoking. The phenotype of the underlying obstructive process in these cases remains under active study, and includes a predominantly airway-centered process and emphysema. For example, exposure to occupational substances has been associated with increased symptoms and worse pulmonary function in α_1-antitrypsin (AAT) deficient individuals, a group at particular risk for emphysema. Furthermore, a cross-sectional study suggested an increased risk of chronic bronchitis, emphysema, and COPD in those exposed to biologic dust. It is likely that an interaction between occupational exposure and cigarette smoking exists, as has been strongly suggested in coke oven exposure. The

Table 5-2: Occupational Exposures Implicated in Causing Chronic Airway Disease

Minerals

- Coal
- Human-made vitreous fibers
- Oil mist
- Portland cement
- Silica
- Quartz

Metals

- Osmium
- Vanadium
- Welding fumes
- Cadmium

Organic dusts

- Cotton
- Grain
- Wood and sawdust

Solvents

Adapted from Balmes, 2005 and Meldrum et al, 2005

diagnostic approach to nonsmoking individuals who develop COPD is more difficult and requires careful attention in assessing the type of exposure, the length of exposure, the use of protective equipment, and the overall hygiene of the workplace.

Risk Factor Reduction
Smoking Cessation

It is evident that smoking cessation is the most important risk modification strategy in patients with COPD. The data presented earlier strongly support successful cessation resulting in preserved lung function, decreased symptoms, and improved mortality. As such, international guideline panels have strongly supported comprehensive smoking cessation programs in the management of COPD.

The effects of nicotine, which is associated with dependence, include an increase in the expression of brain nicotine receptors and a multitude of systemic effects. The result is a combination of disorders that are associated with tobacco addiction, including nicotine dependence and withdrawal. A recent systematic review confirms that few daily smokers spontaneously reduce smoking, and that at any given time, more than 80% of smokers are not seriously planning on quitting. Given these concepts, smoking cessation approaches have generally been multidisciplinary, including: (1) substituting alternate forms of nicotine delivery, (2) administering pharmacologic therapy that ameliorates the effects of withdrawal, and (3) administering behavioral treatments.

Brief counseling from a health-care professional has been reported to result in mildly increased smoking cessation rates. In general, however, a more rigorous, comprehensive approach is required to improve long-term quit rates. The US Agency for Health Care Policy and Research published a sentinel report that established the five steps for smoking cessation known as *The Five A's* (Table 5-3). The use of available resources can improve the approach to smoking cessation, including the use of telephone tobacco quit lines. In November 2004, the Department of Health and Human Services announced a toll-free national number (1-800-QUIT-NOW) to route callers to appropriate services in their region. A recent randomized trial at five Veterans Affairs medical centers confirmed that a telephone-based behavioral

Table 5-3: The 'Five A's' Used to Aid a Patient in Smoking Cessation

1. Ask: Inquire about tobacco use at each office visit. Implement an office-wide system that routinely documents smoking status.

2. Advise: Encourage all patients who smoke to quit smoking. Use a clear, strong, and personalized message to encourage smoking cessation.

3. Assess: Inquire about the patient's willingness to quit. If necessary, provide motivation.

4. Assist: Provide practical counseling and refer to other smoking cessation resources.

5. Arrange: Provide explicit short- and long-term follow-up to evaluate therapies.

Adapted from USPHS report

counseling approach increased the 6-month self-reported abstinence rate compared to standard care (OR 3.50, 95% CI 1.99-6.15).

Comprehensive attempts at smoking cessation generally include some form of nicotine replacement. Table 5-4 provides a general summary of approved products. The variety of available agents allows flexibility in approaching smokers with a variety of smoking habits. Nicotine patches are applied once daily and can be considered 'passive' approaches, while the other products allow the smoker to self-administer a variety of doses. There are several different formulations of patches with differing initial and tapering doses. Their recommended wear time also varies—some are administered every 24 hours, and some can be removed after 16 hours. The main advantage of the patch is compliance. On the other hand, patches may not protect the smoker against acute cravings provoked by smoking-related stimuli. Similarly, data with extended-use patch therapy have yielded inconsistent results in improved long-term abstinence rates.

As noted in Table 5-4, there are numerous forms of 'acute' dosing types of nicotine replacement. These products have the benefit of allowing flexibility in dosing, and can be used for 'breakthrough' cravings. It is important to note that the products should also be used regularly throughout the day, because underdosing is clearly a common problem. The products vary in their administration and nicotine delivery methods. The gum has been available for the longest time and comes in various doses and flavors. The lozenge provides a similar nicotine delivery approach. The inhaler delivers nicotine that is absorbed via the mouth, not the lungs or bronchi. The amount of nicotine absorbed is temperature-dependent, such that use in cold temperatures may decrease the amount delivered. In heavier smokers, the inhaler device appears to be a preferred form of nicotine replacement. The nicotine nasal spray allows delivery of nicotine more rapidly than other acute dosing modalities.

Bupropion (Wellbutrin®, Zyban®) represents a different therapeutic modality approved for smoking cessation and endorsed by the US Clinical Practice Guideline. This antidepressant is chemically unrelated to tricyclic antidepressants or serotonin reuptake inhibitors. One Cochrane meta-analysis reviewed 24 studies and confirmed that long-term abstinence rates were higher with bupropion than with placebo (OR 2.06, 95% CI 1.77-2.40). Limited comparisons with nicotine replacement products have suggested a somewhat greater efficacy with bupropion. In general, this agent is safe if used within the recommended dosages (Table 5-4) and with attention to contraindications (Table 5-5). Because this agent is metabolized hepatically by isoenzyme CYP2B6, it has to be used carefully in patients treated with drugs also metabolized by this enzyme

The most recent agent approved for use in facilitating smoking cessation is varenicline (Chantix™), a partial

Table 5-4: Summary of Quit Rates by Pharmacologic Treatment Type

Treatment	Standard Dose and Duration
Nicotine Replacement	
Transdermal	4-6 weeks of 21 mg + 2 weeks of 14 mg + 2 weeks of 7 mg, 6 weeks of 15 mg + 2 weeks of 10 mg + 2 weeks of 5 mg
Acute delivery formats	
Gum	6-8 weeks of 2 mg, 6-8 weeks of 4 mg
Lozenge	9 per day for 6 weeks followed by 6 week taper
Inhaler	<16 cartridges per day for 12 weeks
Spray	8-40 doses per day for 8 weeks
Non-nicotine	
Bupropion	150 mg daily for 6 days followed with 300 mg daily for 2 more weeks; dose adjustment in elderly, hepatic/renal insufficiency, and in diabetics on oral agent or insulin therapy
Partial nicotinic receptor agonist	
Varenicline (Chantix™)	0.5 mg daily for 3 days then 0.5 mg twice daily for 4 days then 1 mg twice daily

End-of-Treatment Abstinence Rate (%)	6-month Abstinence Rates (%)
15-62	10-54
30-73	19-38
54-81	13-44
46-49	Not reported
28-46	17-35
43-66	24-44
43-60	18-30
40-51	19-23*

*52 weeks

Adapted from Lerman, et al, McRobbie, et al, and Henningfield, et al

Table 5-5: Contraindications and Precautions for Use of Bupropion as a Smoking-Cessation Agent

Contraindications

- Smokers younger than 18 years
- Pregnancy
- Hypersensitivity to bupropion
- Current or previous seizure disorder
- Tumor of the central nervous system
- Current or previous diagnosis of bulimia or anorexia nervosa
- Severe hepatic cirrhosis
- Concomitant use of bupropion and monoamine oxidase inhibitors
- History of bipolar disorder
- Withdrawal from alcohol or benzodiazepines

Precautions

- Risk-benefit assessment recommended in individuals at risk for seizures including:
  - Medications that lower seizure threshold (antidepressants, antipsychotics, antimalarials, quinolones, sedating antihistamines, systemic corticosteroids, theophylline, tramadol [Ultracet®, Ultram®])
  - Current use of stimulants or anorectics
  - Alcohol abuse
  - History of head injury

Adapted from McRobbie et al

agonist of the nicotinic receptors. This agent selectively binds to the $\alpha_4\beta_2$-receptor, the receptor subtype that has generally been associated with the addictive (reinforcing) effects of nicotine. The available clinical data suggest that the medication is efficacious and is associated with few adverse events. In comparisons with bupropion, varenicline was associated with better quit rates. No data are available in patients younger than 18 years of age.

Given the limited benefit of individual agents, numerous investigators have combined drugs to optimize smoking cessation rates. Combination of transdermal nicotine replacement with acute nicotine delivery has resulted in modest incremental benefit. The combination of nicotine replacement with bupropion appears to yield somewhat better short- and long-term results, although the data are inconsistent. Combination therapy data are most consistently favorable for the combination of behavioral approaches with pharmacotherapy. Combination of varenicline with nicotine replacement in a limited number of patients appears to be associated with greater side effects.

Reduction in Occupational Exposure

Prevention of occupational-induced chronic airway disease involves primary, secondary, and tertiary prevention strategies. Primary strategies involve a hierarchy of exposure controls, including elimination, engineering controls, administrative controls, and the use of personal protective equipment. Secondary prevention strategies emphasize screening to identify early disease in patients at risk for a detrimental host response to chronic exposure, with hope to minimize exposure and prevent progression to severe disease. Tertiary prevention requires identification of individuals with established COPD in whom appropriate therapy is instituted in an effort to prevent progressive, permanent disease. This may involve removal from exposure or, at the very least, reduction of the intensity of exposure. Complementary to all of these approaches is appropriate screening in the at-risk workplace, including both medical screening

73

and exposure monitoring. Useful techniques include sensitive, symptom-based questionnaires to identify symptoms highly suggestive of exposure. In addition, judicious use of spirometric screening may prove quite useful. An analysis of the Third Annual NHANES survey suggested that industries at risk included rubber, plastics, leather manufacturing, utilities, building services, textile manufacturing, the armed forces, food products manufacturing, chemical, petroleum, coal manufacturing, and construction.

Conclusion

Chronic obstructive pulmonary disease represents a syndrome resulting from an accentuated inflammatory response to inhaled substances in susceptible individuals. The majority of cases can be related to cigarette smoking with a significant minority related to inhalation of various occupational and environmental substances. Smoking cessation has been demonstrated to preserve lung function, decrease respiratory symptoms, and improve mortality. As such, this intervention is a key component of COPD management schema. Occupational and other environmental exposures have become increasingly recognized, although data regarding environmental controls of exposure are slowly accumulating.

Suggested Readings

An LC, Zhu SH, Nelson DB, et al: Benefits of telephone care over primary care for smoking cessation: a randomized trial. *Arch Intern Med* 2006;166:536-542.

Anthonisen NR, Connett JE, Kiley JP, et al: Effect of smoking intervention and the use of an inhaled anticholinergic bronchodilator on the rate of decline of FEV1. The Lung Health Study. *JAMA* 1994;272:1497-1505.

Anthonisen NR, Connett JE, Murray RP: Smoking and lung function of Lung Health Study participants after 11 years. *Am J Respir Crit Care Med* 2002;166:675-679.

Anthonisen NR, Skeans MA, Wise RA, et al: The effects of a smoking cessation intervention on 14.5-year mortality: a randomized clinical trial. *Ann Intern Med* 2005;142:233-239.

Balmes JR: Occupational contribution to the burden of chronic obstructive pulmonary disease. *J Occup Environ Med* 2005;47: 154-160.

Balmes J, Becklake M, Blanc P, et al: American Thoracic Society Statement: Occupational contribution to the burden of airway disease. *Am J Respir Crit Care Med* 2003;167:787-797.

Behrendt CE: Mild and moderate-to-severe COPD in nonsmokers: Distinct demographic profiles. *Chest* 2005;128:1239-1244.

Celli BR, Halbert RJ, Nordyke RJ, et al: Airway obstruction in never smokers: results from the Third National Health and Nutrition Examination Survey. *Am J Med* 2005;118:1364-1372.

Celli BR, MacNee W, ATS/ERS Task Force: Standards for the diagnosis and treatment of patients with COPD: a summary of the ATS/ERS position paper. *Eur Respir J* 2004;23:932-946.

Connett JE, Murray RP, Buist AS, et al: Changes in smoking status affect women more than men: results of the Lung Health Study. *Am J Epidemiol* 2003;157:973-979.

Foulds J: The neurobiological basis for partial agonist treatment of nicotine dependence: varenicline. *Int J Clin Pract* 2006;60:571-576.

Global Strategy for Diagnosis, Management, and Prevention of COPD. 2006 Update.

Gonzales D, Rennard SI, Nides M, et al: Varenicline, an alpha4beta2 nicotinic acetylcholine receptor partial agonist, vs sustained-release bupropion and placebo for smoking cessation: a randomized controlled trial. *JAMA* 2006;296:47-55.

Hnizdo E, Sullivan PA, Bang KM, et al: Association between chronic obstructive pulmonary disease and employment by industry and occupation in the US population: a study of data from the Third National Health and Nutrition Examination Survey. *Am J Epidemiol* 2002;156:738-746.

Hu Y, Chen B, Yin Z, et al: Increased risk of chronic obstructive pulmonary diseases in coke oven workers: interaction between occupational exposure and smoking. *Thorax* 2006;61:290-295.

Hughes JR, Carpenter MJ: The feasibility of smoking reduction: an update. *Addiction* 2005;100:1074-1089.

Hughes JR, Stead LF, Lancaster T. Antidepressants for smoking cessation. In: *The Cochrane Library*, issue 4, Chichester, UK, John Wiley & Sons Ltd, 2004. Available at: http://www.mrw.interscience. wiley.com. Accessed November 8, 2006.

Ingersoll KS, Cohen J: Combination treatment for nicotine dependence: state of the science. *Subst Use Misuse* 2005;40:1923-1943, 2043-2048.

Jorenby DE, Hays JT, Rigotti NA, et al: Efficacy of varenicline, an alpha4beta2 nicotinic acetylcholine receptor partial agonist, vs placebo or sustained-release bupropion for smoking cessation: a randomized controlled trial. *JAMA* 2006;296:56-63.

Lerman C, Patterson F, Berrettini W: Treating tobacco dependence: state of the science and new directions. *J Clin Oncol* 2005; 23:311-323.

Lundback B, Lindberg A, Lindstrom M, et al: Not 15 but 50% of smokers develop COPD?-Report from the Obstructive Lung Disease in Northern Sweden Studies. *Respir Med* 2003;97:115-122.

Matheson MC, Benke G, Raven J, et al: Biological dust exposure in the workplace is a risk factor for chronic obstructive pulmonary disease. *Thorax* 2005;60:645-651.

McRobbie H, Lee M, Juniper Z: Non-nicotine pharmacotherapies for smoking cessation. *Respir Med* 2005;99:1203-1212.

Meldrum M, Rawbone R, Curran AD, et al: The role of occupation in the development of chronic obstructive pulmonary disease (COPD). *Occup Environ Med* 2005;62:212-214.

Menezes AM, Perez-Padilla R, Jardim JR, et al: Chronic obstructive pulmonary disease in five Latin American cities (the PLATINO study): a prevalence study. *Lancet* 2005;366:1875-1881.

Rennard SI, Vestbo J: COPD: the dangerous underestimate of 15%. *Lancet* 2006;367:1216-1219.

Simmons MS, Connett JE, Nides MA, et al: Smoking reduction and the rate of decline in FEV(1): results from the Lung Health Study. *Eur Respir J* 2005;25:1011-1017.

The Tobacco Use and Dependence Clinical Practice Guideline Panel, Staff, and Consortium Representatives: A clinical practice guideline for treating tobacco use and dependence. A US Public Health Service report. *JAMA* 2000;283:3244-3254.

Tonstad S, Tonnesen P, Hajek P, et al: Effect of maintenance with varenicline on smoking cessation. A randomized controlled trial. *JAMA* 2006;296:64-71.

Varkey AB: Chronic obstructive pulmonary disease in women: exploring gender differences. *Curr Opin Pulm Med* 2004;10:98-103.

Chapter 6

Management of Stable COPD

The guidelines of the Global Initiative for Chronic Obstructive Lung Disease (GOLD) (Figure 6-1) workshop and the American Thoracic Society (ATS)/ European Respiratory Society (ERS) (Figure 6-2) recommend that the effective management of stable chronic obstructive pulmonary disease (COPD) include the following components: (1) assessing and monitoring the disease; (2) reducing risk factors; (3) managing the disease; and (4) managing exacerbations. The major goals of therapy outlined by this approach include relief of symptoms; prevention of progression of the disease; improvement of exercise tolerance; improvement of health status; prevention and treatment of complications; prevention and treatment of exacerbations; and reduction of mortality. The diagnostic and prevention components are examined in other chapters of this book. The overall approach to management is characterized by a stepwise increase in treatment based on the severity of the disease and/or the patient's symptoms, and includes a patient education section. The treatment options that we have now can reduce or abolish symptoms, increase exercise capacity, and reduce the number of exacerbations.

Bronchodilator Therapy

Most patients with COPD have a component of airflow obstruction that is responsive to bronchodilators.

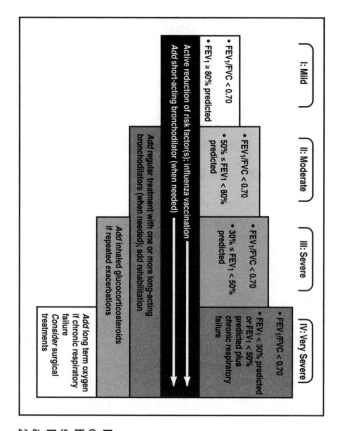

Figure 6-1: Recommendation for patient therapy based on GOLD COPD stages. Global Strategy for Diagnosis, Management, and Prevention of COPD. 2006 Update.

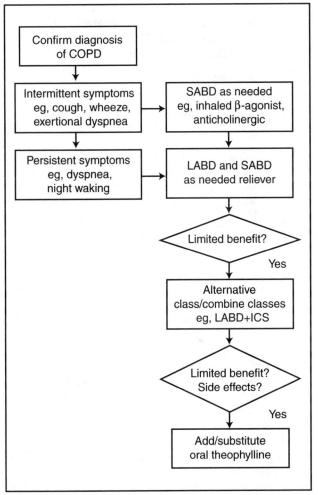

Figure 6-2: Algorithm of treatment options for COPD based on the ATS/ERS guidelines. ICS=inhaled corticosteroids; LABD=long-acting bronchodilators; SABD=short-acting bronchodilators. Reprinted with permission from Celli BR, MacNee W, *Eur Respir J* 2004;23:932-946.

Table 6-1: Steps for Appropriate Use of Metered-Dose Inhaler Bronchodilator

- Remove cap
- Shake inhaler
- Hold inhaler upright
- Tilt head back 10° to 15°
- Position inhaler 2-4 cm in front of open mouth (patients with poor hand-to-breath coordination should consider use of extension devices or spacers)
- Begin inhalation and then activate inhaler
- Inhale slowly and deeply to total lung capacity
- Hold breath for 5-10 seconds
- Exhale slowly through nose
- Inhale one puff; wait 3-5 minutes between inhalation of subsequent puffs

Although the amount of reversibility achieved may vary, any improvement in airflow will be critically important in managing these patients. Furthermore, recent studies have demonstrated that there are other beneficial physiologic effects of bronchodilators, including a decrease in patients' hyperinflation (decrease in lung volumes), improved exercise tolerance, improved quality of life, and a decrease in the frequency of exacerbations. The guidelines recommend two classes of bronchodilator medications, inhaled anticholinergics and β_2-adrenergic receptor agonists, for the management of symptomatic COPD. These two classes of bronchodilators differ in their mechanism of effect, in that inhaled anticholinergics decrease bronchoconstriction and glandular secretions via the inhibition of acetylcholine, while β_2-adrenergic receptor agonists induce bronchodilatation by acting on the β_2-adrenergic receptors located in the smooth muscle of the airway. Tables 6-1 and 6-2 summarize the steps in the appropriate use of these medications as well as their onset of action and dosing frequency in COPD. Another class of bronchodilators, the methylxanthines, are available but their use for the treatment of COPD remains controversial because of their increased risk of adverse effects.

Short-acting β_2-agonists

The regular use vs as-needed use of short-acting β_2-agonist therapy for airflow obstruction in patients with COPD has generated considerable controversy. Studies have primarily examined regular vs as-needed short-acting β-agonists used in asthma, but little is known about any benefit in COPD. Several randomized trials in asthma have shown that there was no difference in the use of regular albuterol compared to as-needed therapy in the rate of morning peak flows or exacerbations. Furthermore, recent reports have linked the regular use of short-acting β_2-agonists with increased cardiac-related complications in COPD patients. Cook et al tested the hypothesis that patients with COPD may derive no benefit from regular vs as-needed inhaled short-acting β_2-agonist therapy; these investigators conducted a randomized, concealed, double-blind, placebo-controlled, crossover trial to evaluate the efficacy of regular vs as-needed albuterol (Proventil®, Ventolin®). All patients received ipratropium bromide (Atrovent®) at 20 μg per puff in 2 puffs 4 times daily, beclomethasone (Beclovent®, nasal inhalers) at 250 μg per puff or equivalent corticosteroids dose, and open-label inhaled albuterol as needed. This study showed that patients used twice as much active albuterol in the regular-use period (mean 8.07 puffs of coded and 4.68 puffs of open-label medication, a total of 12.75 puffs daily), than during the as-needed period (mean

Table 6-2: Onset of Action and Dosing Frequency of Commonly Used Inhalers in COPD

Drug	Inhaler Dose (μg)	Dosing Frequency
Short-acting β_2-agonists		
Albuterol (Proventil®, Ventolin®)	90-180 200, DPI, HFA	q 4-6 h
Short-acting anticholinergics		
Ipratropium bromide (Atrovent®) (Atrovent ® HFA)	20-40 MDI, HFA 17-34 MDI 18-36 MDI	q 4-6 h
Long-acting β_2-agonists		
Salmeterol (Serevent®)	50 DPI	q 12 h
Formoterol (Foradil®)	12-24 DPI	q 12 h
Arformoterol tartrate (Brovana™)	25 μg b.i.d.	q 12 h
Long-acting anticholinergics		
Tiotropium (Spiriva®)	18 DPI	q 24 h

6.34 puffs of open-label albuterol daily). Despite greater short-acting β_2-agonist use, patients showed similar results during treatment and control periods of all outcomes. These investigators concluded that COPD patients used twice as much short-acting inhaled β_2-agonist in a regular-use

Drug	Inhaler Dose (μg)	Dosing Frequency
Inhaled corticosteroids		
Budesonide (Pulmicort®)*	100, 200 DPI, inhaled solution	q 12 h
Fluticasone propionate (Flovent®)*	50-500 DPI	
Mometasone (Asmanex®)*	220/440 DPI	q 12 h
Combination therapy		
Fluticasone propionate + salmeterol (Advair Diskus®)	100/50*, 250/50, 500/50* DPI 45/21,* 115/21,* 230/21* HFA	q 12 h
Formoterol + budesonide* (Symbicort®)	4.5/80 μg and 4.5/160 μg DPI	

*Approved by the FDA only for asthma.
DPI = dry power inhaler; HFA = hydrofluoroalkane;
MDI = metered-dose inhaler

period without physiologic or clinical benefits, compared to patients who took the drug on an as-needed basis.

There are limited data on the effects of short-acting β_2-agonists on quality-of-life outcomes for patients with COPD, other than changes in lung function. Clinical studies have shown that treatment with albuterol (salbutamol) significantly improves dyspnea and overall health status in patients with severe COPD compared with oral theophylline; the studies have also shown that additive treatment with albuterol for patients taking other bronchodilators is beneficial. Thus, the COPD guidelines primarily recommend short-acting β_2-agonists as *rescue* medications in patients with COPD.

Long-acting β_2-agonists (LABA)

The first phase of maintenance therapy in COPD involves treatment with one or more long-acting bronchodilators. Long-acting β_2-agonists, such as salmeterol (Serevent®) and formoterol (Foradil®), have been shown to be effective in patients with stable COPD. These drugs produce prolonged bronchodilation effects (up to 12 hours), decrease nocturnal symptoms, and improve the patient's quality of life. Long-acting β_2-agonists are not indicated for acute exacerbations of COPD. Several clinical studies have shown that salmeterol significantly improved pulmonary function as well as daily and nighttime symptoms compared with placebo and ipratropium (Figure 6-3). During treatment with salmeterol, forced expiratory volume in 1 second (FEV_1) improved significantly and patients experienced significantly less breathlessness as measured by the 6-minute walk distance test. The results of clinical studies also indicate that salmeterol can significantly decrease the frequency of COPD exacerbations (Figure 6-4).

Current treatment guidelines support the regular treatment of COPD with LABAs to improve health status and quality of life. Salmeterol and formoterol treatment have been shown to enhance quality of life for patients with COPD. These studies have shown that twice-daily treatment significantly improves quality of life, as assessed by the St. George's Respiratory Questionnaire (SGRQ) and by the SF-36 health survey. Studies have also shown that LABAs result in superior effects on quality of life com-

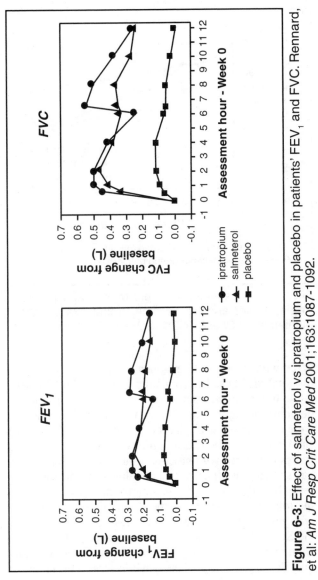

Figure 6-3: Effect of salmeterol vs ipratropium and placebo in patients' FEV_1 and FVC. Rennard, et al: *Am J Resp Crit Care Med* 2001;163:1087-1092.

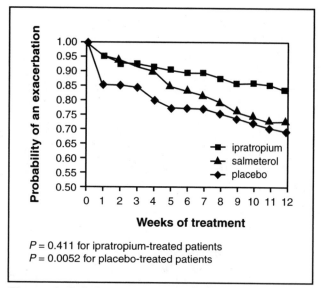

Figure 6-4: Salmeterol vs ipratropium and placebo: Kaplan-Meier analysis of time to first exacerbation. Mahler, et al: *Chest* 1999;115:957-965.

pared with ipratropium treatment—significantly improving total SGRQ scores compared with placebo ($P<0.01$), while treatment with ipratropium (40 µg q.i.d.) failed to demonstrate significant effects on quality of life (findings were comparable with placebo). Studies have shown that salmeterol (12 µg b.i.d.) significantly improved SGRQ scores compared with baseline values, and another study has shown that higher doses of salmeterol (50 µg b.i.d.) result in clinically significant improvements (>4 U) in both the total SGRQ score and the impact domain compared with placebo. Comparative study results, as assessed by the SF-36, have also shown that salmeterol (50 µg b.i.d.) significantly improved quality of life compared with theophylline treatment (goal theophylline serum concentration

10 to 20 µg/mL), for the domains of physical functioning (P=0.02), health perception (P=0.03), and social functioning (P=0.004). Furthermore, because LABAs provide prolonged efficacy (>12 h) compared with short-acting β_2-agonists (4 to 6 hours), LABAs may be more convenient for the patient, which may promote medication adherence and, consequently, may improve COPD management.

The US Food and Drug Administration (FDA) recently approved arformoterol tartrate (Brovana™) solution, a long-acting β_2-agonist for long-term maintenance treatment in patients with COPD. Arformoterol tartrate is the first long-term β_2-agonist to be developed for use with a nebulizer. In phase III studies, patients treated with arformoterol for 12 months demonstrated a significant improvement in FEV_1 compared with placebo.

Anticholinergic Agents

Inhaled anticholinergic drugs such as ipratropium have been used for more than 30 years and have been shown to be safe and effective. A limitation of anticholinergics is their necessary frequent use (4 times daily). The use of a fixed combination of short-acting β_2-agonist and ipratropium is helpful in the management of COPD. The bronchodilator effect achieved by using this combination therapy is superior to that achieved with either agent alone, and may be used if warranted by the severity of the patient's condition. This combination therapy reduces the need for high doses of short-acting β_2-agonist, and reduces the toxicity associated with this therapy.

The once-daily anticholinergic tiotropium (Spiriva®) was recently approved for use in stable COPD. Tiotropium is an anticholinergic bronchodilator maintenance treatment with a long duration of action, attributed to slow dissociation from airway M_3 muscarinic receptors that allow once-daily dosing. Placebo-controlled studies have shown that once-daily inhalation with tiotropium 18 µg significantly improves airflow and FEV_1 over 24 hours in patients with

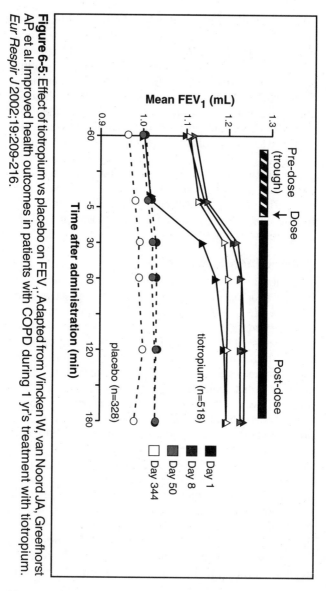

Figure 6-5: Effect of tiotropium vs placebo on FEV$_1$. Adapted from Vincken W, van Noord JA, Greefhorst AP, et al: Improved health outcomes in patients with COPD during 1 yr's treatment with tiotropium. *Eur Respir J* 2002;19:209-216.

COPD, and these benefits were consistently maintained over the year (Figure 6-5). Furthermore, these and other studies have consistently shown that tiotropium significantly improves dyspnea, decreases exacerbations, and improves exercise tolerance leading to improvements in HR quality of life. Adverse events were comparable with placebo, except for dry mouth, whose incidence with tiotropium was 16% vs 2.7% with placebo ($P<0.05$). Similar results were reported by Vincken et al in long-term studies with this drug. These data show that tiotropium is an effective, once-daily bronchodilator that reduces dyspnea and exacerbation frequency, and improves health status. Based on these observations of lower rates of exacerbations and hospitalizations, a prospective 6-month, placebo-controlled trial was conducted at 26 Veterans Administration centers, comparing tiotropium to placebo. This study showed a significant reduction in exacerbation frequency in patients treated with tiotropium compared to those who received placebo.

No other intervention, with the exception of smoking cessation, has been proven to decrease the rate of FEV_1 decline in COPD. Recent data suggest that tiotropium bromide may possibly change the clinical course of the disease. In an analysis of two identical 1-year, randomized, double-blind studies involving 535 COPD patients, tiotropium (18 µg once daily) increased trough FEV_1 by 120 mL at the end of the trial, while treatment with ipratropium (40 µg 4 times daily) was associated with a 30 mL reduction in trough FEV_1 ($P<0.001$). Anzueto et al performed a post hoc analysis using data from 921 ambulatory COPD patients who participated in the two 1-year, randomized, controlled registration trials of tiotropium. Patients reached steady state on tiotropium therapy within 8 days. The change in trough FEV_1 from day 8 to day 344 was -12.4 mL/year in the tiotropium group and -58.0 mL/year in the placebo group ($P=0.005$).

The sustained improvement in lung function seen during these 1-year studies with tiotropium suggests that tiotropium may slow the decline in lung function over time and subsequently change the clinical course of the disease. A longer-term study named UPLIFT is underway to examine these potential effects.

Methylxanthines

Treatment of COPD with long-acting formulations of methylxanthines (eg, aminophylline and theophylline) remains controversial because of their small therapeutic window and their well-documented adverse effects. They are, however, still often used to treat COPD patients who are unresponsive to β_2-agonists and to treat acute exacerbations. Aminophylline is generally administered intravenously for the treatment of respiratory failure. Studies have shown that theophylline treatment, particularly when given in combination with other bronchodilators, improves quality of life for patients with COPD. It should be stated, however, that theophylline is generally regarded as a third-line treatment option for COPD, and theophylline serum concentrations must be carefully monitored to ensure clinical efficacy and safety. GOLD guidelines recommend inhaled bronchodilator therapy over theophylline because of theophylline's recognized possible adverse effects, such as atrial and ventricular arrhythmias and grand mal convulsions.

Corticosteroid Therapy

Airway inflammation has been documented in patients with chronic airflow obstruction. Given the impact of COPD on patients' general health and well-being, and the cost associated with treating acute exacerbations, which often require inpatient care, treatment regimens that avoid hospitalization are desired by patients, physicians, and third-party payers. A recent observational study of more than 22,000 elderly COPD patients reported that the use of inhaled corticosteroids (ICS) was independently associated with a decreased risk of readmission and mortality. Clinical studies have shown that COPD patients treated with ICS may have better health-related quality of life, lower rates of exacerbation (Figure 6-6), fewer respiratory symptoms, and lower risk of rehospitalization or death within the first year after an initial hospitalization. Several investigators have shown that the combination of an ICS with a long-acting β_2-agonist (LABA) has a significant reduction of risk of hospitalization.

There are six ICS options available for the treatment of asthma and COPD: beclomethasone dipropionate (Beclovent®), budesonide (Pulmicort®), flunisolide (AeroBid®), fluticasone propionate (Flovent®), mometasone furoate (Asmanex®), and triamcinolone acetonide (Azmacort®) (Table 6-2). GOLD and ATS/ERS guidelines recommend ICSs to treat patients with severe-to-very-severe COPD or with acute exacerbations. Clinical study results have shown that ICS therapy reduced the rate of COPD exacerbations, which led to an improved health status, and have also shown that certain ICS agents enhance quality of life for patients with COPD. After 4 months of treatment with fluticasone propionate (500 μg b.i.d.), patients who continued to receive the drug for an additional 6 months experienced significant improvements in total SGRQ scores (+2.48, 95% CI [confidence interval]: 0.37-4.58), as well as in symptom (+4.58, 95% CI: 1.05-8.10) and activity (+4.64, 95% CI: 1.60-7.68) domains, compared with patients who discontinued the treatment and received placebo instead. In addition, a 3-year study assessing the long-term effects of fluticasone propionate in COPD showed that treatment (500 μg b.i.d.) not only significantly reduced the rate of deterioration in total SGRQ scores compared with placebo ($P<0.004$), but also resulted in significant improvements in physical function ($P<0.005$), energy/vitality ($P<0.02$), and mental health domains of the SF-36 health survey ($P<0.005$). Furthermore, the SGRQ total score of patients treated with fluticasone propionate deteriorated at a rate 59% slower than that of patients receiving placebo treatment.

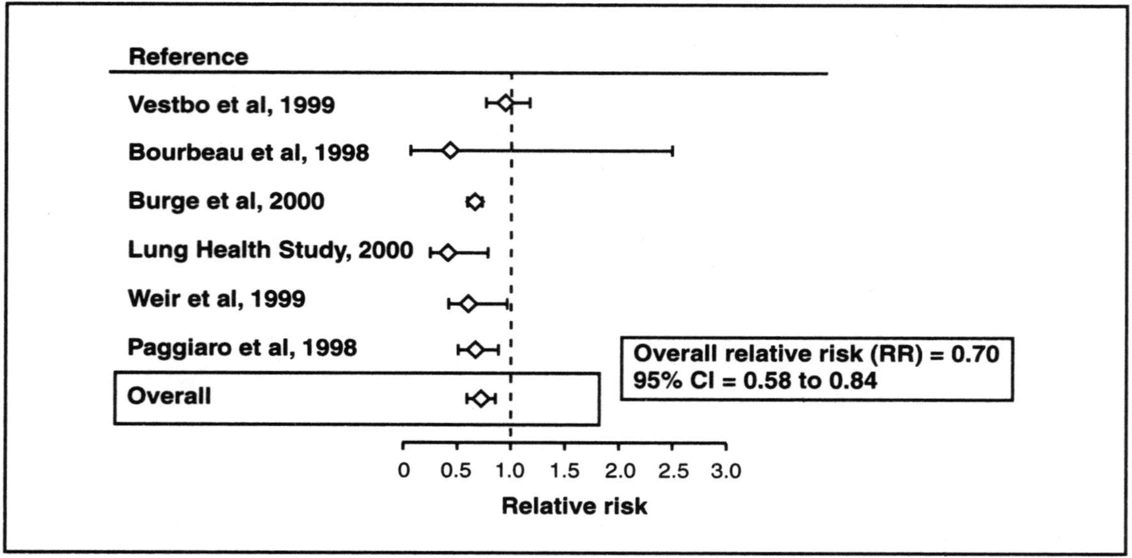

Figure 6-6: Relative risk of exacerbations in COPD patients treated with ICS: a meta-analysis. Alsaeedi et al, *Am J Med* 2002;113:59-65.

However, not all clinical studies assessing the effects of ICS therapies on quality of life have demonstrated positive or consistent results. In a 4-year study by van Schayck et al, treatment with beclomethasone dipropionate did not result in any significant improvements in quality of life compared with salbutamol or ipratropium treatment, as measured by the Inventory of Subjective Health (ISH) and Nottingham Health Profile (NHP), however, clinically significant improvements (>4 U) in the SGRQ symptom score were observed in another study by John et al after 12 weeks of treatment with beclomethasone dipropionate (400 µg b.i.d., HFA formulation [QVAR®]) compared with placebo. That study also showed a slight, although not significant, improvement in total SGRQ score. Interestingly, significant improvements in lung function were observed by van Schayck et al after beclomethasone dipropionate treatment despite the lack of any improvement in quality of life, which further demonstrates the weak correlation between clinical outcomes and an individual's perceived quality of life. However, it should be stated that the lack of significant quality-of-life results could be due to the medications or instruments used in these studies. Neither the ISH nor the NHP were specifically designed to evaluate COPD patient outcomes.

Inhaled corticosteroids have been shown to decrease acute exacerbation of COPD. Some studies have failed to demonstrate a role for ICSs in speeding up symptom resolution, but these trials have not been designed to answer this question. A recently published prospective, randomized trial comparing high-dose nebulized budesonide (2 mg q 6 h for 72 h) with prednisone (30 mg twice daily for 72 h), demonstrated no difference between active treatments, with both being superior to placebo in recovery of FEV_1.

Oral or intravenous corticosteroid therapies have limited value in patients with COPD. There is mounting evidence that a short course of oral corticosteroids is a good predictor of long-term response to inhaled medication. Current guidelines do not recommend their use.

Combination Therapy

ICS and LABA Combination. COPD guidelines also recommend LABAs given in combination with ICSs for patients with advanced COPD who remain symptomatic despite bronchodilator therapy. Data with inhaled fixed combinations of LABAs and ICSs have shown an improvement in spirometry, dyspnea, and reduction in the frequency of exacerbations. In a clinical trial, 691 patients with COPD received the combination of fluticasone propionate and salmeterol (500 µg/50 µg), salmeterol (50 µg), fluticasone propionate (500 µg), or placebo twice daily for 24 weeks. At the end of the trial, lung function significantly improved with all treatments compared with placebo ($P<0.05$); however, the combination of fluticasone propionate and salmeterol (Advair Diskus®) provided significantly greater improvement compared with either treatment alone ($P<0.05$). The combination also significantly improved dyspnea compared with fluticasone propionate ($P=0.033$), salmeterol ($P<0.001$), and placebo ($P<0.0001$). In this trial, health status and symptoms were also significantly improved. Similar results were observed in another trial with fluticasone propionate and salmeterol combination (250 µg/50 µg) (Figure 6-7). Another combination of ICS and LABA, budesonide and formoterol (Symbicort®), has been studied. In a 1-year trial, patients with COPD received budesonide/formoterol 320 µg/9 µg, budesonide 400 µg, formoterol 9 µg, or placebo. Patients receiving budesonide/formoterol 320 µg/9 µg had fewer exacerbations, a prolonged time to first exacerbation, and maintained higher FEV_1, compared with placebo. There was also a reduction of the mean rate of severe exacerbations (ie, those requiring the use of oral steroids and/or antibiotics and/or hospitalization caused by respiratory symptoms) significantly more than placebo and formoterol ($P<0.05$).

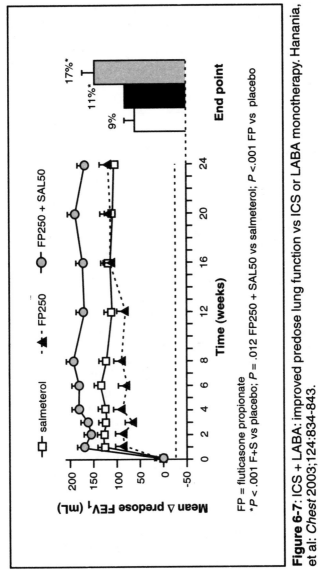

Figure 6-7: ICS + LABA: improved predose lung function vs ICS or LABA monotherapy. Hanania, et al: *Chest* 2003;124:834-843.

Table 6-3: TORCH Study Design

- Aged 40-80 years
- FEV_1 <60% predicted
- Reversibility <10% predicted normal to 400 µg albuterol

Run-in

2 weeks

*All treatments administered via the Diskus® device.
Vestbo J, TORCH Study Group: The TORCH (towards a revolution in COPD health) survival study protocol. Modified from *Eur Respir J* 2004;24:206-210.

The combination also improved HR quality of life. The combination of budesonide/formoterol was more effective than either of the individual treatments alone. Another trial with the combination budesonide/formoterol showed significant decrease in all symptom scores and improved quality of life compared with placebo.

Several retrospective analyses of ICS use in COPD patients have examined the association between ICS and survival. In a review of 2,620 residents of Ontario, Canada, who were 65 years of age and older, and those hospitalized for COPD at least once, those who received ICS within 90 days of hospital discharge had a substantially lower adjusted relative risk (RR 0.74, 95% CI, 0.71-0.78) for repeat hospitalization or death compared with those who did not receive ICS. In a study based in England, COPD patients who were regular users of salmeterol and/or fluticasone propionate had significantly better 3-year survival than patients not using these medications. A recent report from two different managed care organiza-

	Planned number of patients
Advair Diskus® 500/50* b.i.d.	1,510
Fluticasone propionate 500 b.i.d.	1,510
Salmeterol 50 b.i.d.	1,510
Placebo	1,510
3 years	6,040

tions from different parts of the United States found that patients who used ICS, LABA, or ICS plus LABA had better survival than patients who used only short-acting bronchodilators. Furthermore, the survival effect was preserved even after adjustment for other clinical factors likely to affect survival, including age, disease severity, comorbid diseases, and smoking history.

The impact of combination therapy (fluticasone propionate/salmeterol) on patients' mortality, frequency of exacerbations, and long-term effects also has recently been reported. The Towards a Revolution in COPD Health (TORCH) study is the first study to prospectively investigate the potential for combination therapy (fluticasone propionate/salmeterol) to affect survival in patients with COPD (Table 6-3). The TORCH study is a 3-year, multicenter, randomized, double-blind, parallel group, placebo-controlled study. Approximately 6,100 patients were randomized into four study groups: placebo, salmeterol, fluticasone propionate (500 µg), and fluticasone

Table 6-4: Impact of Fluticasone and Salmeterol on Mortality in COPD

Comparison	HR	95% CI
Fluticasone/ salmeterol vs placebo*	0.825	0.68-1.00
Salmeterol vs placebo	0.88	0.73-1.06
Fluticasone vs placebo	1.06	0.89-1.27

CI=confidence interval; HR=hazards ratio
*Adjusted for 2 interim analyses.

Calverley PM, et al: Program and abstracts of the 2006 European Respiratory Society Annual Meeting (Poster E311).

propionate/salmeterol (500 μg/50 μg). The primary end point was the reduction in all-cause mortality, comparing fluticasone propionate/salmeterol with placebo (Table 6-4). Secondary end points included COPD morbidity (rate of exacerbations) and quality-of-life assessment. Preliminary results have been presented at two international meetings. Table 6-5 enumerates the results of the primary analyses on mortality. In the first analysis, the absolute reduction in 3-year, all-cause mortality was 2.6%, while the relative risk was 17.5% (P=0.052 after adjustment for two interim analyses). No differences were seen in secondary comparisons of fluticasone and salmeterol compared with placebo. A secondary analysis using Cox proportional hazards modeling supported the primary effect of combination therapy on mortality compared with placebo (HR=0.811, 95% CI: 0.67-0.98, P=0.031). No significant interaction was noted when these analyses were repeated by baseline FEV_1 by GOLD stage, smoking

Table 6-5: Effect of Fluticasone/Salmeterol vs Placebo on All-Cause Mortality at 3 Years

		Placebo (n=1,524)	Fluticasone/ salmeterol (n=1,533)
Probability of death by 3 years (%)*		15.2	12.6

	HR	95% CI	P
Unadjusted	0.820	(0.677, 0.993)	0.041
Adjusted**	0.825	(0.681, 1.002)	0.052

*Estimated 17.5% reduction in risk of dying at any time in 3 years; 2.6% absolute risk reduction

**Adjusted for 2 interim analyses.

Calverley PM, et al: Program and abstracts of the 2006 European Respiratory Society Annual Meeting (Poster E311).

status, age, gender, or body mass index (BMI). Secondary comparisons are shown in Table 6-6. It is evident that combination therapy was associated with a 25% reduction in moderate-to-severe exacerbations compared with placebo; less impressive, but statistically significant, decreases were noted with fluticasone and salmeterol alone compared with placebo. Analyses of SGRQ scores and pulmonary function also confirmed beneficial effects over the duration of the study for the combination agent. The combination of fluticasone and salmeterol was generally well tolerated with no evidence of HPA (hypothalmic/pituitary/adrenal) axis, cardiac events, or bone toxicity; there was an increase in investigator-reported pneumonias without a difference in the total number of lower respiratory tract infections. These data suggest that pharmacologic therapy in COPD can result in survival, health status, exacerbation reduction, and physiologic benefits. This is the first prospective study

Table 6-6: Impact of Fluticasone and Salmeterol on Health Status, Pulmonary Function, and Exacerbations

Secondary end point	Fluticasone/salmeterol vs placebo HR (95% CI)
Moderate-to-severe exacerbations* (RR)	0.75 (0.69, 0.81) $P<0.0001$
SGRQ total score	-3.1 (-4.1, -2.1) $P<0.0001$
Postbronchodilator FEV_1 (mL)	92 (75,108) $P<0.001$

*Moderate=antibiotics and/or systemic corticosteroids; Severe=hospitalization

in which the primary end point was patient survival. The study results showed that in patients with moderate-to-severe COPD (stages II to IV), the treatment with ICS and LABA combination therapy could decrease mortality. More studies will be needed to verify these findings.

β_2-agonist/Anticholinergics Combination

Combining bronchodilators with varying durations of effect and mechanisms of action may also benefit patients with COPD, as bronchodilator combination therapy has been shown to increase the degree of bronchodilation more than bronchodilator monotherapy. Also, combining bronchodilators has demonstrated adverse event profiles that are equal to or less than those observed for each component when administered alone. Studies have demonstrated the positive impact of bronchodilator combination therapies that combine a β_2-agonist with an anticholinergic. Bronchodilator combination therapies are also recommended

Fluticasone/salmeterol vs salmeterol HR (95% CI)	Fluticasone/salmeterol vs fluticasone HR (95% CI)
0.88 (0.81, 0.95) $P=0.002$	0.91 (0.84, 0.99) $P=0.024$
-2.2 (-3.1, -1.2) $P<0.0001$	-1.2 (-2.1, -0.2) $P=0.017$
50 (34, 67) $P<0.001$	44 (28, 61) $P<0.001$

Celli BR, et al: Program and abstracts of the 2006 European Respiratory Society Annual Meeting (Poster E312).

by GOLD and ATS/ERS guidelines to achieve additional improvements in health status.

Although clinical studies have shown that LABA and ipratropium combination therapies improve lung function to greater degrees than administration of each monotherapy, these studies failed to demonstrate any additional improvements in quality of life, as assessed with the Chronic Respiratory Disease Questionnaire (CRDQ). Other studies, however, have shown that ipratropium, given in combination with a LABA, significantly improves quality of life (as assessed by the SGRQ) compared with ipratropium given in combination with albuterol for patients with COPD.

Long-acting β_2-agonist treatment, given in combination with tiotropium, has also been shown to be clinically effective for the treatment of COPD. Long-term and large-scale studies are needed to fully evaluate the effectiveness of this combination therapy.

Other Treatments
Mucolytic Agents

A 1998 meta-analysis suggested that oral mucolytic agents such as N-acetylcysteine or iodinated glycerol reduced the frequency of acute exacerbations in COPD patients. Oral mucolytic agents reduced exacerbations by 22% in patients who had an average of 5.5 exacerbations per year. A more typical patient with COPD having 2 to 3 exacerbations per year would, however, expect to reduce exacerbations by less than one by taking mucolytic agents daily for 2 to 3 years. No effect on rate of decline of FEV_1 was seen. A more recent meta-analysis on the effect of oral N-acetylcysteine revealed similar results in terms of a decrease in COPD exacerbations in patients treated for 12 to 24 weeks. In addition, a recently published update of Poole's Cochrane analysis confirmed the beneficial results of N-acetylcysteine, and determined that the number of patients needed to treat for one patient to have no exacerbations during the study period was six. A study in Switzerland suggested that therapy with N-acetylcysteine was cost effective. The mechanism by which N-acetylcysteine reduces COPD exacerbations is unclear, but may be related to enhanced macrophage activity, which would help defend against mucosal infections. N-Acetylcysteine therapy should be considered in patients with more than five exacerbations per year. Treatment with mucolytic agents has failed to show any benefits in patients during an acute exacerbation.

Leukotriene-Receptor Antagonists

There is no evidence supporting the use of leukotriene-receptor antagonists in COPD. These agents block the actions of the cysteinyl leukotrienes that have an important role in asthma, but have not been shown to have a demonstrable effect in COPD. The available leukotriene-receptor antagonists have no effect on leukotriene B_4 (LTB_4), which has a role in the pathogenesis of chronic bronchitis and COPD. Future studies will examine the effects of specific LTB_4 antagonists in COPD.

Table 6-7: Oxygen Delivery Devices, Flow Rate, and Approximate FiO$_2$

Device	Flow rate (L/min)	Approximate FiO$_2$
Nasal cannula	1 - 10	0.24 - 0.5
Face mask	8 - 12	0.35 - 0.65
Venturi mask	2 - 10	0.24 - 0.45
Partial rebreathing mask	6 - 10	0.3 - 0.6
Nonrebreathing mask	6 - 12	0.4 - 0.9
Misty-Ox®	6 - 30	0.4 - 0.9

FiO$_2$ = fraction of inspired oxygen

Supplemental Oxygen Therapy

Long-term oxygen therapy (LTOT) reverses hypoxemia, prevents hypoxia, and has been shown to improve life expectancy in patients with COPD. Patients whose disease is stable on a full medical regimen, with PaO$_2$ <55 mm Hg (corresponding to a SaO$_2$ <88%), should receive long-term oxygen therapy. Patients with PaO$_2$ between 55 and 59 mm Hg (SaO$_2$ 89%) and who exhibit signs of tissue hypoxia, such as pulmonary hypertension, cor pulmonale, erythrocytosis, edema from right heart failure, or impaired mental status, should also receive LTOT. Patients with desaturation only during exercise or sleep might be candidates for oxygen therapy, specifically under those conditions. Table 6-7 summarizes oxygen delivery devices, flow rate, and approximate FiO$_2$. Figure 6-8 shows the ATS/ERS LTOT algorithm.

Vaccination

For more details on the role of vaccinations in stable COPD, see Chapter 8.

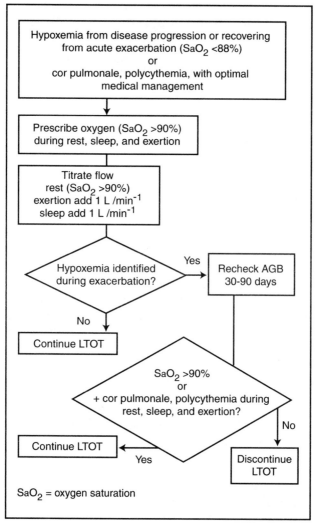

Figure 6-8: ATS/ERS Long-term oxygen treatment (LTOT) algorithm. Celli BR, MacNee W: *Eur Respir J* 2004;23: 932-946.

Suggested Readings

Anzueto A, Tashkin D, Menjoge S, et al: One-year analysis of longitudinal changes in spirometry in patients with COPD receiving tiotropium. *Pulm Pharmacol Ther* 2005;18:75-81.

Backman R, Hellström PE: Formoterol and ipratropium bromide for treatment of patients with chronic bronchitis. *Curr Ther Res* 1985;38:135-140.

Barnes PJ: Chronic obstructive pulmonary disease. *N Engl J Med* 2000;343:269-280.

Bellia V, Foresi A, Bianco S, et al: Efficacy and safety of oxitropium bromide, theophylline and their combination in COPD patients: a double-blind, randomized, multicentre study (BREATH Trial). *Respir Med* 2002;96:881-889.

Boyd G, Morice AH, Pounsford JC, et al: An evaluation of salmeterol in the treatment of chronic obstructive pulmonary disease (COPD). *Eur Respir J* 1997;10:815-821.

Briggs DD Jr, Doherty DE: Long-term pharmacologic management of patients with chronic obstructive pulmonary disease. *Clin Cornerstone* 2004;(suppl 2):S17-S28.

British Thoracic Society guidelines for the management of chronic obstructive pulmonary disease. *Thorax* 1997;52:S1-S28. Available at: http://thorax.bmj.com. Accessed November 8, 2006.

Brusasco V, Hodder R, Miravitlles M, et al: Health outcomes following treatment for six months with once daily tiotropium compared with twice daily salmeterol in patients with COPD. *Thorax* 2003;58:399-404. Erratum in *Thorax* 2005;60:105.

Burge PS, Calverley PM, Jones PW, et al: Randomised, double-blind, placebo-controlled study of fluticasone propionate in patients with moderate to severe chronic obstructive pulmonary disease: the ISOLDE trial. *BMJ* 2000;320:1297-1303.

Calverley PM, Boonsawat W, et al: Maintenance therapy with budesonide and formoterol in chronic obstructive pulmonary disease. *Eur Respir J* 2003;22:912-919.

Casaburi R, Mahler DA, Jones PW, et al: A long-term evaluation of once-daily inhaled tiotropium in chronic obstructive pulmonary disease. *Eur Respir J* 2002;19:217-224.

Celli B, Calverley PM, Anderson JA, et al: The TORCH (Towards a Revolution in COPD Health) Study: Fluticasone propionate/salmeterol improves health status, reduces exacerbations, and improves lung function over 3 years. 2006 European Respiratory Society Annual Meeting (Poster E312).

Celli BR, MacNee W, ATS/ERS Task Force: Standard for the diagnosis and treatment of patients with COPD: a summary of the ATS/ERS position paper. *Eur Respir J* 2004;23:932-946.

Cheer SM, Scott LJ: Formoterol: a review of its use in chronic obstructive pulmonary disease. *Am J Respir Med* 2002;1:285-300.

Cook D, Guyatt G, Wong E, et al: Regular versus as-needed short-acting inhaled beta-agonist therapy for chronic obstructive pulmonary disease. *Am J Respir Crit Care Med* 2001;163:85-90.

Decramer M, Celli B, et al: Clinical trial design considerations in assessing long-term functional impacts of tiotropium in COPD: The Uplift Trial. *J COPD* 2004;1:303-312.

Disse B, Speck GA, Rominger KL, et al: Tiotropium (Spiriva): mechanistical considerations and clinical profile in obstructive lung disease. *Life Sci* 1999;64:457-464.

Dorinsky PM, Reisner C, Ferguson GT, et al: The combination of ipratropium and albuterol optimizes pulmonary function reversibility testing in patients with COPD. *Chest* 1999;115:966-971.

Dougherty JA, Didur BL, Aboussouan LS: Long-acting inhaled beta 2-agonists for stable COPD. *Ann Pharmacother* 2003;37:1247-1255.

Duffy N, Walker P, Diamantea F, et al: Intravenous aminophylline in patients admitted to hospital with non-acidotic exacerbations of chronic obstructive pulmonary disease: a prospective randomised controlled trial. *Thorax* 2005;60:713-717.

Fabbri L, Pauwels RA, Hurd SS: Global Strategy for the Diagnosis, Management and Prevention of Chronic Obstructive Pulmonary Disease: GOLD Executive Summary updated 2003. *COPD* 2004;1:105-141; discussion 103-104.

Global Strategy for Diagnosis, Management, and Prevention of COPD. 2006 Update.

Hanania NA, Darken P, Horstman D, et al: The efficacy and safety of fluticasone propionate (250 microg)/salmeterol (50 microg) combined in the Diskus inhaler for the treatment of COPD. *Chest* 2003;124:834-843.

Karpel JP, Pesin J, Greenberg D, et al: A comparison of the effects of ipratropium bromide and metaproterenol sulfate in acute exacerbation of COPD. *Chest* 1990;98:835-839.

Littner MR, Ilowite JS, Tashkin DP, et al: Long-acting broncho-dilation with once-daily dosing of tiotropium (Spiriva) in stable chronic obstructive pulmonary disease. *Am J Respir Crit Care Med* 2000;161(4 pt 1):1136-1142.

Lotvall J: Pharmacology of bronchodilators used in the treatment of COPD. *Respir Med* 2000;94(suppl E):S6-S10.

Lung Health Study Research Group: Effect of inhaled triamcinolone on the decline of pulmonary function in chronic obstructive pul-monary disease. *N Engl J Med* 2000;343:1902-1909. Available at: http://content.nejm.org. Accessed November 8, 2006.

Mahler DA, Donohue JF, Barbee RA, et al: Efficacy of salmeterol xinafoate in the treatment of COPD. *Chest* 1999;115:957-965.

Mahler DA, Wire P, Horstman D, et al: Effectiveness of fluticasone propionate and salmeterol combination delivered via the Diskus device in the treatment of chronic obstructive pulmonary disease. *Am J Respir Crit Care Med* 2002;166:1084-1091.

Mapel D, Hurley JS, Roblin I, et al: Survival of COPD patients using inhaled corticosteroids and long-acting beta agonists. *Respir Med* 2006;100:595-609.

Moayyedi P, Congleton J, Page RL, et al: Comparison of nebulised salbutamol and ipratropium bromide with salbutamol alone in the treatment of chronic obstructive pulmonary disease. *Thorax* 1995;50:834-837.

Niewoehner DE, Erbland ML, Deupree RH, et al: Effect of systemic glucocorticoids on exacerbations of chronic obstructive pulmonary disease. Department of Veterans Affairs Cooperative Study Group. *N Engl J Med* 1999;340:1941-1947.

Pauwels RA, Buist AS, Calverley PM, et al: Global strategy for the diagnosis, management, and prevention of chronic obstructive pulmonary disease. NHLBI/WHO Global Initiative for Chronic Obstructive Lung Disease (GOLD) Workshop summary. *Am J Respir Crit Care Med* 2001;163:1256-1276.

Pauwels RA, Lofdahl CG, Laitinen LA, et al : Long-term treatment with inhaled budesonide in persons with mild chronic obstructive pulmonary disease who continue smoking. European Respiratory Society Study on Chronic Obstructive Pulmonary Disease. *N Engl J Med* 1999;340:1948-1953.

Rice KL, Leatherman JW, Duane PG, et al: Aminophylline for acute exacerbations of chronic obstructive pulmonary disease. A controlled trial. *Ann Intern Med* 1987;107:305-309.

Sin DD, Tu JV: Inhaled corticosteroids and the risk of mortality and readmission in elderly patients with chronic obstructive pulmonary disease. *Am J Respir Crit Care Med* 2001;164:580-584.

Soriano JB, Vestbo J, Pride NB, et al: Survival in COPD patients after regular use of fluticasone propionate and salmeterol in general practice. *Eur Respir J* 2002;20:819-825.

Suissa S: Effectiveness of inhaled corticosteroids in chronic obstructive pulmonary disease: immortal time bias in observational studies. *Am J Respir Crit Care Med* 2003;168:49-53.

Szafranski W, Cukier A, Ramirez A, et al: Efficacy and safety of budesonide/formoterol in the management of chronic obstructive pulmonary disease. *Eur Respir J* 2003;21:74-81.

Tashkin DP, Ashutosh K, Blecker ER, et al: Comparison of the anticholinergic bronchodilator ipratropium bromide with metaproterenol in chronic obstructive pulmonary disease. A 90-day multicenter study. *Am J Med* 1986;8:81-90.

Van Noord JA, Bantje TA, Eland ME, et al: A randomised controlled comparison of tiotropium and ipratropium in the treatment of chronic obstructive pulmonary disease. The Dutch Tiotropium Study Group. *Thorax* 2000;55:289-294.

Vestbo J, Sorensen T, Lange P, et al: Long-term effect of inhaled budesonide in mild and moderate chronic obstructive pulmonary disease: a randomised controlled trial. *Lancet* 1999;353:1819-1823.

Vestbo J: The TORCH (towards a revolution in COPD health) survival study protocol. TORCH Study Group. *Eur Respir J* 2004; 24:206-210.

ZuWallack RL, Mahler DA, Reilly D, et al: Salmeterol plus theophylline combination therapy in the treatment of COPD. *Chest* 2001;119:1661-1670.

Chapter 7

Nonpharmacologic Therapy

The therapeutic approach to chronic obstructive pulmonary disease (COPD) includes pharmacologic and nonpharmacologic interventions. The latter include a wide range of options, such as long-term oxygen therapy (LTOT), pulmonary rehabilitation, nutritional support, and surgical therapies.

Long-term Oxygen Therapy

Long-term oxygen therapy is one of the few therapeutic interventions that positively affects survival in patients with COPD. This conclusion is based on the results of randomized trials, which documented improved survival in COPD patients who met strict criteria and were treated with oxygen. The British Medical Research Council study demonstrated that hypoxemic patients treated with 15 hours/day of oxygen (including during sleep) experienced improved survival. Similarly, the Nocturnal Oxygen Therapy Trial found improved survival in hypoxemic patients treated with continuous oxygen (average 19 hours/day) compared with those treated with oxygen for approximately 12 hours/day (including during sleep). It thus appears that continuous oxygen therapy is appropriate for patients who meet criteria for advanced hypoxemia, although a plausible mechanism for the improvement in survival is unclear. In addition, the benefits of oxygen therapy are optimal if supplementation lasts for more than 15 hours/day.

Data suggest that LTOT improves exercise, sleep, and cognitive performance in selected patients. The role of oxygen therapy in patients with less-severe hypoxemia remains unclear. In studies of patients with milder daytime hypoxemia, LTOT has not shown dramatic benefits, although all studies were limited by low power. More data are required to better define the role of oxygen therapy with milder hypoxemia, including exercise-induced desaturation.

Determining which patients will benefit from LTOT requires an accurate assessment of oxygenation. Measurement of arterial blood gases is the optimal approach to determining the need for and level of oxygen supplementation. Measurement of oxygen saturation by pulse oximetry is adequate for trending. Using classically established criteria, Figure 6-8 enumerates the current indications for LTOT. These criteria should be confirmed during a time of clinical stability. Reassessment of oxygenation status after an exacerbation is recommended, although the optimal timing remains controversial. For example, several groups have confirmed that anywhere between one third to one half of patients who initially meet the criteria for LTOT no longer do so after reevaluation 1 to 2 months later.

Pulmonary Rehabilitation

Pulmonary rehabilitation has been defined as "...a multidisciplinary program of care for patients with chronic respiratory impairment that is individually tailored and designed to optimize physical and social performance and autonomy." Systematic reviews have demonstrated that pulmonary rehabilitation improves exercise capacity, decreases exertional breathlessness, improves health status, and decreases health-care use. These beneficial effects have been found in patients with disease severities ranging from mild-to-severe COPD. Improvement in symptoms and exercise capacity has been demonstrated to persist with long-term maintenance. COPD patients with chronic respiratory impairment who, despite optimal medical management, are persistently symptomatic, have reduced exercise tolerance, or experience a restriction in activities, are appropriate candidates for pulmonary rehabilitation. The patient evaluation should include an interview, a detailed medical evaluation, diagnostic testing, psychosocial assessment, and the setting of appropriate goals.

Pulmonary rehabilitation should be a multimodal, therapeutic intervention, individualized and targeted to the patient's physical and social function. Elements should include education, psychosocial/behavioral intervention, institution of appropriate respiratory and chest physiotherapy techniques, exercise training, ventilatory muscle training in selected patients, and clear outcome assessment. A key element of this comprehensive approach is exercise training, which should be tailored to the individual's physical abilities and interests as well as institutional resources and environment. Exercise programs can be prescribed to include lower-extremity exercise, upper-extremity exercise, or both. Finally, improvement in functional status has been reported with inpatient, outpatient, and home rehabilitation approaches.

Nutrition

Weight loss has been a well-recognized complication in COPD patients for many years. Similarly, many investigators have confirmed that weight loss is associated with increased mortality in COPD. Increased investigation has confirmed abnormalities not only in body weight but also in body composition. For example, fat-free mass has been demonstrated to be a more accurate predictor of mortality, as has midthigh muscle cross-sectional area. Data strongly suggest that loss of muscle mass is particularly important in COPD patients. The nature of these findings is under intense investigation but may reflect sequelae of the systemic, inflammatory response known to occur in COPD, altered dietary intake, increased work of breathing, and altered energy metabolism of skeletal muscle.

Given the importance of nutritional status in COPD, numerous investigative groups have assessed the impact of intense nutritional support on outcomes in these patients. A recent Cochrane review of randomized trials suggested little change in anthropometric measures or functional exercise capacity. In contrast, a combination of nutritional supplementation with exercise training and/or anticatabolic agents may be a novel approach. Controlled trials are ongoing to define the role of such a therapeutic approach in COPD patients.

Volume Reduction
Surgical

For the past 50 years surgical approaches to ameliorate symptoms in COPD patients have been studied, with lung volume reduction surgery (LVRS) being the most successful. The surgical approach to LVRS has included median sternotomy, standard thoracotomy, and video-assisted procedures. Laser ablation has fallen out of favor because of a high complication rate and improvements in other modalities. In general, greater improvement with bilateral than with unilateral procedures has been reported. Since the earliest reports, numerous studies have confirmed significant short-term, mean improvements in spirometry, lung volume, exercise capacity, breathlessness, and health status. Unfortunately, significant heterogeneity in response has been reported, with a significant proportion of patients experiencing little improvement in spirometry, even in the short term.

Given the heterogeneity in response, much has been written about identifying which patients should and which should not be considered for surgery. Pulmonary function testing has proven instrumental in identifying optimal candidates. The National Emphysema Treatment Trial (NETT) identified subgroups of patients at particularly high risk of surgical mortality after bilateral LVRS (Figure 7-1). High-risk patients included those with a postbronchodilator FEV_1 ≤20% predicted and a diffusing capacity of the lung for carbon monoxide (DLCO) ≤20% predicted. Imaging of the chest has also proven highly predictive of outcome. The NETT demonstrated that high-resolution computed tomography (CT) of the chest, in combination with physiologic variables, identified good and poor candidates for LVRS. The physiologic variables included results of oxygen-supplemented maximal cycle ergometry. A threshold of 40% of the baseline, maximal achieved workload identified a clear break point in mortality for the overall study group. This threshold corresponded to a workload of 25 watts for females and 40 watts for males.

These thresholds, in conjunction with CT data, allowed a clear separation of low-risk patients into distinct categories. These groups were associated with identifiable differences in mortality and functional outcome as described by changes in the St. George's Respiratory Questionnaire (SGRQ), a disease-specific instrument commonly used to assess health-related quality of life in COPD, and by exercise capacity (Figure 7-1 and Table 7-1). Table 7-2 lists potential indications and contraindications for the same populations.

Bronchoscopic

Novel techniques that allow selective bronchoscopic lung volume reduction have become available. These techniques produce localized areas of atelectasis and lung volume reduction. Those under study include those in which a one-way valve is placed into hyperinflated, emphysematous segments, and those in which an occlusive plug is placed in selected segments. These approaches have been tested in small case series with inconsistent benefits, although improvement in dynamic hyperinflation in select patients treated with bronchoscopic placement of valves has been documented. Controlled trials are ongo-

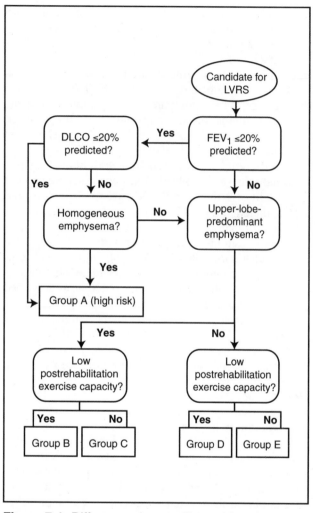

Figure 7-1: Differences in mortality and functional outcomes in COPD disease-specific groups. Martinez FJ, Flaherty KR, Iannettoni MD: Patient selection for LVRS. *Chest Surg Clin N Am* 2003;13:669-685.

ing and should shed further light on the potential role of such a therapeutic intervention.

Transplantation

Lung transplantation is an accepted surgical option in carefully selected COPD patients. The optimal patients for such an intervention remain difficult to identify because it is inherently challenging to make definitive statements about mortality risk in these patients. In fact, long-term survival is possible in patients with advanced disease. Conflicting data have been published regarding survival benefits of lung transplantation in COPD. Median survival for the COPD recipient population is approximately 5 years, and 10-year survival is achieved by only 20% to 25% of patients. Therefore, many have advocated that lung transplantation should be viewed as a life-enhancing rather than life-extending procedure for COPD patients. Lung transplantation should be offered to patients with advanced disease who remain extremely ill despite maximal pharmacologic therapy and rehabilitation, and who are willing to accept the associated risks. Table 7-3 lists potential general and disease-specific guidelines for identifying patients who may be candidates for lung transplantation. Figure 7-2 provides a potential approach to decision making for the patient with COPD referred for transplantation.

The optimal transplant procedure for COPD patients remains controversial, with single lung transplantation (SLT) being the most commonly performed. Functional outcomes following SLT and bilateral lung transplantation (BLT) have been extensively investigated, with both producing improved pulmonary function and exercise capacity. Some groups have reported that BLT may provide superior functional results and lower mortality. An additional consideration is the pros and cons of the two procedures with regard to organ availability. Whether SLT or BLT more efficiently uses limited resources requires additional investigation.

Table 7-1: Results of Bilateral LVRS Compared to Medical Therapy in Patients With Severe Emphysema

Patients	90-Day Mortality		P Value
	LVRS	Medical Therapy	
Group A	20/70 (28.6)	0/70 (0)	<0.001
Group B	4/139 (2.9)	5/151 (3.3)	1.00
Group C	6/206 (2.9)	2/213 (0.9)	0.17
Group D	7/84 (8.3)	0/65 (0)	0.02
Group E	11/109 (10.1)	1/111 (0.9)	0.003

Patients	Improvement in Exercise Capacity*			
	LVRS	Medical Therapy	Odds Ratio	P Value
Group A	4/58 (7)	1/48 (2)	3.48	0.37
Group B	25/84 (30)	0/92 (0)	—	<0.001
Group C	17/115 (15)	4/138 (3)	5.81	0.001
Group D	6/49 (12)	3/41 (7)	1.77	0.50
Group E	2/65 (3)	2/59 (3)	0.90	1.00

Values in parentheses indicate percentages.
Groups A-E refer to the patients defined in Figure 7-2.

*Increase in the maximal workload of more than 10W from the patient's postrehabilitation baseline value (24 months after randomization)

†Risk ratio for total mortality in surgically vs medically treated patients during a mean follow-up of 29.2 months.

Total Mortality			
LVRS	Medical Therapy	Risk Ratio[†]	P Value
42/70	30/70	1.82	0.06
26/139	51/151	0.47	0.005
34/206	39/213	0.98	0.70
28/84	26/65	0.81	0.49
27/109	14/111	2.06	0.02

Improvement in Health-related Quality of Life[‡]			
LVRS	Medical Therapy	Odds Ratio	P Value
6/58 (10)	0/48 (0)	—	0.03
40/84 (48)	9/92 (10)	8.38	<0.001
47/115 (41)	15/138 (11)	5.67	<0.001
18/49 (37)	3/41 (7)	7.35	0.001
10/65 (15)	7/59 (12)	1.35	0.61

[‡] Improvement in the health-related quality of life was defined as a decrease in score on the St. George's Respiratory Questionnaire of more than 8 points (on a 100-point scale) from the patient's postrehabilitation baseline score (24 months after randomization).

Adapted from Fishman A, Martinez F, Naunheim K, et al: A randomized trial comparing lung-volume-reduction surgery with medical therapy for severe emphysema. *N Engl J Med* 2003;348:2059-2073 and Martinez FJ, Flaherty KR, Iannettoni MD: Patient selection for lung volume reduction surgery. *Chest Surg Clin N Am* 2003;12:669-685.

Table 7-2: Potential Indications and Contraindications for LVRS

Parameter	Indications
Clinical	• Age <75 yr
	• Clinical picture consistent with emphysema
	• Dyspnea despite maximal medical treatment, pulmonary rehabilitation
	• Former smoker (>6 mo)
	• Requiring <20 mg prednisone/d
Physiologic	• FEV_1 after bronchodilator <45% predicted
	• Hyperinflation – TLC >100% predicted – RV >150%
	• PaO_2 >45 mm Hg
	• $PaCO_2$ <60 mm Hg
	• Postrehabilitation 6 minute walk distance >140 m
	• Low postrehabilitation maximal achieved cycle ergometry watts
Imaging	• *CXR*—Hyperinflation
	• *CT*—High-resolution CT confirming severe emphysema, upper-lobe predominance

Adapted from http//www.thoracic.org/copd and Martinez FJ, Chang A: Surgical therapy for chronic obstructive pulmonary disease. *Sem Respir Crit Care Med* 2005;26:167-191.
FEV_1=forced expiratory volume in 1 second

Contraindications

- Age >75-80 yr
- Comorbid illness that increases surgical mortality
- Clinically significant coronary artery disease
- Pulmonary hypertension
  (PA systolic >45, PA mean >35 mm Hg)
- Surgical constraints:
  – Previous thoracic procedure
  – Pleuradesis
  – Chest wall deformity
- FEV_1 ≤20% predicted and DLCO ≤20% predicted
- ↑ inspiratory resistance

- Homogeneous emphysema and FEV_1 <20% predicted
- Non-upper-lobe predominant emphysema and
  high postrehabilitation cycle ergometry maximal
  achieved wattage

Table 7-3: General and Disease-specific Selection Guidelines for Candidate Selection for Lung Transplantation in COPD Patients

General Selection Guidelines
Relative Contraindications

- Age limits
  - Heart-lung transplant ~55 yr
  - Double-lung transplant ~60 yr
  - Single-lung transplant ~65 yr
- Poorly treated or untreated, symptomatic osteoporosis
- Oral corticosteroids >20 mg/d prednisone
- Ideal body weight <70% or >130%
- Psychosocial problems
- Requirement for invasive mechanical ventilation
- Colonization with fungi or atypical mycobacteria

COPD Disease-specific Criteria

- FEV_1 <20% to 25% predicted
- PCO_2 >7.3 kPa (55 mm Hg)
- Homogeneous emphysema distribution
- Pulmonary hypertension

Conclusion

The optimal therapeutic approach to COPD includes both pharmacologic and nonpharmacologic approaches. The latter include many options. The best defined include LTOT in hypoxemic patients, pulmonary rehabilitation in persistently symptomatic patients, nutritional supple-

Absolute Contraindications

- Severe musculoskeletal disease affecting the thorax
- Substance addiction within previous 6 months
- Dysfunction of extrathoracic organ, particularly renal dysfunction
- Human immunodeficiency virus infection
- Active cancer within 2 years, except basal or squamous cell carcinoma of skin
- Hepatitis B antigen positivity
- Hepatitis C with biopsy-proven evidence of liver disease

Adapted from http://www.thoracic.org/copd and Martinez FJ, Chang A: Surgical therapy for chronic obstructive pulmonary disease. *Semin Respir Crit Care Med* 2005;26:167-191.

mentation in selected individuals, and surgical therapies. LVRS has proven survival and palliative benefit in carefully selected emphysema patients. Lung transplantation likely has a role in a small subset of the most severely ill COPD patients.

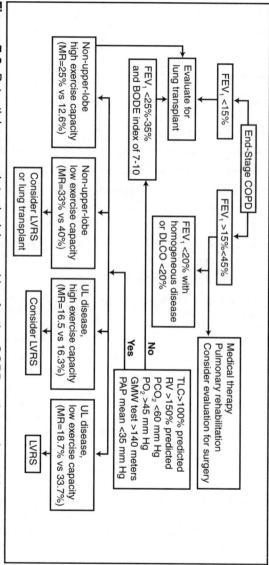

Figure 7-2: Potential approach to decision making for the COPD patient referred for lung transplantation. Nathan SD: Lung transplantation: disease-specific considerations for referral. *Chest* 2005;127:1006-1016.

Suggested Readings

American Thoracic Society: Pulmonary rehabilitation-1999. *Am J Respir Crit Care Med* 1999;159(5 pt 1):1666-1682.

Benditt JO: Surgical therapies for chronic obstructive pulmonary disease. *Respir Care* 2004;49:53-61; discussion 61-63.

Celli BR, MacNee W, ATS/ERS Task Force: Standards for the diagnosis and treatment of patients with COPD: a summary of the ATS/ERS position paper. *Eur Respir J* 2004;23:932-946.

Crockett AJ, Cranston JM, Moss JR, et al: Domiciliary oxygen for chronic obstructive pulmonary disease. *Cochrane Database Syst Rev* 2000;CD001744.

Ferreira IM, Brooks D, Lacasse Y, et al: Nutritional supplementation for stable chronic obstructive pulmonary disease. *Cochrane Database Syst Rev* 2005;CD000998.

Fishman A, Martinez F, Naunheim K, et al: A randomized trial comparing lung-volume-reduction surgery with medical therapy for severe emphysema. *N Engl J Med* 2003;348:2059-2073.

Global Strategy for Diagnosis, Management, and Prevention of COPD. 2006 Update.

Hopkinson NS, Toma TP, Hansell DM, et al: Effect of bronchoscopic lung volume reduction on dynamic hyperinflation and exercise in emphysema. *Am J Respir Crit Care Med* 2005;171:453-460.

MacNee W: Prescription of oxygen: still problems after all these years. *Am J Respir Crit Care Med* 2005;172:517-518.

Martinez FJ, Chang A: Surgical therapy for chronic obstructive pulmonary disease. *Semin Respir Crit Care Med* 2005;26:167-191.

Martinez FJ, Flaherty KR, Iannettoni MD: Patient selection for lung volume reduction surgery. *Chest Surg Clin N Am* 2003;12:669-685.

Nathan SD: Lung transplantation: disease-specific considerations for referral. *Chest* 2005;127:1006-1016.

Salman GF, Mosier MC, Beasley BW, et al: Rehabilitation for patients with chronic obstructive pulmonary disease: meta-analysis of randomized controlled trials. *J Gen Intern Med* 2003;18:213-221.

Schols A: Nutritional modulation as part of the integrated management of chronic obstructive pulmonary disease. *Proc Nutr Soc* 2003;62:783-791.

Chapter 8

Acute Exacerbations of COPD

The American Thoracic Society/European Respiratory Society (ATS/ERS) and the Global Initiative for Chronic Obstructive Lung Disease (GOLD) have proposed to define exacerbations of chronic obstructive pulmonary disease (COPD) as "events in the natural course of the disease characterized by a change in the patient's baseline dyspnea, cough and/or sputum beyond day-to-day variability sufficient to warrant a change in management." These organizations have also proposed this classification of severity: level I is treated at home; level II requires hospitalization; and level III leads to respiratory failure. Various factors probably contribute to the acute exacerbations of COPD, including industrial pollutants, allergens, sedatives, congestive heart failure (CHF), and infections (viral and bacterial). The cause of an exacerbation may be multifactorial, so that viral infection or levels of air pollution may exacerbate the existing inflammation in the airways, which in turn may predispose the patient to secondary bacterial infections. Bacterial infections are believed to play a part in one half to two thirds of exacerbations.

Magnitude of the Problem

Acute exacerbations of COPD are a common cause of morbidity and mortality in this patient population. Acute exacerbation of COPD is associated with frequent visits to physicians. Patients with these conditions account for more than 14 million physician office visits and 500,000 hospitalizations annually. COPD is the second leading cause of work disability (back pain is the leading cause) and the third most common diagnosis for home-care services. It has been estimated that the cost of treating COPD is $24 billion each year, including hospitalization costs and days off from work. The frequency with which patients experience exacerbations can be used to grade the severity of chronic bronchitis as a disease process. United States data indicate that in 1998, COPD and related infectious exacerbations were responsible for an estimated 14.2 million ambulatory visits, 1.4 million emergency department visits, and 662,000 hospitalizations. Significant numbers of hospitalized patients with acute exacerbations have modifiable risk factors including having had an influenza vaccination, or oxygen supplementations, smoking, and occupational exposures.

Several studies have tried to identify the risk factors associated with mortality from acute exacerbation. The Study to Understand Prognosis and Preferences for Outcomes and Rates of Treatment (SUPPORT) enrolled 1,016 patients who had severe acute exacerbation of COPD at hospital admission due to respiratory infections, including pneumonia (48%), CHF (26%), worsening respiratory failure due to lung cancer (3.3%), pulmonary emboli (1.4%), and pneumothorax (1%). The 180-day mortality rate was 33%, and the 2-year mortality rate was 49% (Figure 8-1).

Significant predictors of mortality include acute physiology and chronic health evaluation (APACHE III) score, body mass index, age, functional status 2 weeks before admission, lower ratio of PO_2 to FiO_2, CHF, serum albumen

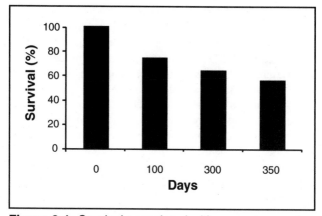

Figure 8-1: Survival associated with severe exacerbation of COPD.

level, cor pulmonale, lower activities of daily living scores, and lower scores on the Duke Activity Status Index. This study also reported that only 25% of patients were both alive and able to report a good, very good, or excellent quality of life 6 months after discharge.

In another large prospective cohort study, patients were admitted to intensive care units (ICUs) with COPD-related respiratory failure. The in-hospital mortality rate, 23.8%, was predicted by number of hospital days before transfer to the ICU, and by the nonrespiratory component of the APACHE III score. A separate analysis to identify true predictors of 180-day mortality included acute physiologic score, age, and hospital days before transfer to the ICU. A separate analysis to identify true predictors of 180-day mortality included acute physiologic score, old age, and more hospital days before transfer to the ICU. Activities of daily living were also significant predictors of univariate analysis.

In a recent report of a cohort of 101 patients with moderate-to-severe COPD (mean forced expiratory volume in 1 second [FEV_1] 41.9% predicted), closely followed up for 2.5

years, increased dyspnea and colds at onset of exacerbation were associated with prolonged recovery times. Recovery was incomplete in a significant proportion of COPD exacerbations. Patients with frequent exacerbations (median 3 to 8/year) experienced a significantly poorer quality of life as measured by the St. George's Respiratory Questionnaire (SGRQ). Factors that predicted frequent exacerbations were the number of exacerbations in the previous year and a history of bronchitic symptoms (cough and sputum production), though lung function was not predictive (Figure 8-2).

Exacerbations also have a major impact on the patients' quality of life. COPD patients are twice as likely as the general population to rate their health as being fair or poor, nearly twice as likely to report recent limitations in their usual activities, and many report frequent visits to their physicians.

COPD is characterized by an accelerated decline in lung function and by periods of acute exacerbation. The frequency of acute exacerbations has been demonstrated to have a significant impact on the decline of lung function. The Lung Health Study (LHS) data showed that smokers with frequent self-reported lower respiratory tract illnesses resulting in physician visits had a significantly increased rate of decline of FEV_1. Recently, Donalson et al reported that patients with frequent exacerbations had a significantly faster decline in FEV_1 and a peak expiratory flow rate (PEFR) of -40.1 mL/year (n=16) and -2.9 L/min/year (n=46). Among people with infrequent exacerbations, FEV_1 changed by -32.1 mL/year (n=16) and PEFR by -0.7 L/min/year (n=63). Those with frequent exacerbations also had the greater decline in FEV_1 if allowance was made for smoking status (Figure 8-3). This study showed that exacerbation frequency is an important determinant of decline in lung function in COPD. Strategies for preventing COPD exacerbations may have an important impact on the natural course of this disease and on the morbidity and mortality of these patients.

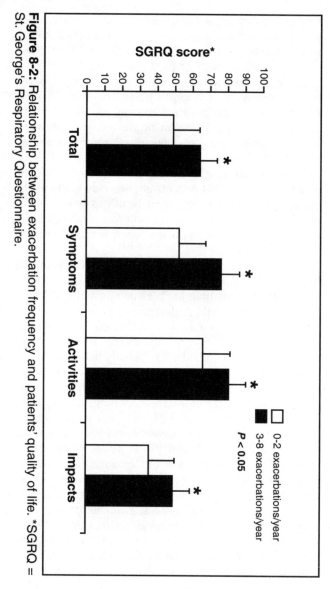

Figure 8-2: Relationship between exacerbation frequency and patients' quality of life. *SGRQ = St. George's Respiratory Questionnaire.

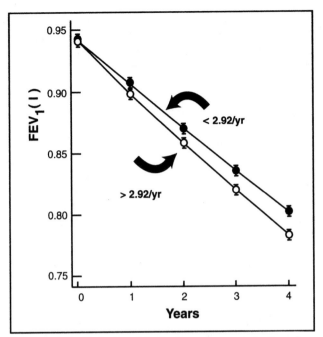

Figure 8-3: Relationship between exacerbation frequency and the rate of lung function decline.

The cost of treating acute exacerbation of COPD is high, not only because of its economic impact, but also because of the increase in morbidity and early mortality. Chronic obstructive pulmonary disease in the United States annually accounts for 16,000,367 office visits, 500,000 hospitalizations, and $18 billion in direct health-care costs.

Relapse

Despite treatment with antibiotics, bronchodilators, and corticosteroids, up to 28% of patients discharged from the emergency department with acute exacerbations of COPD have recurrent symptoms within 14 days, and 17% relapse and require hospitalization. Physicians' ability to identify patients who are at risk for relapse should improve decisions about hospital admissions and follow-up appointments. The risk factors for exacerbation of relapses are: low pretreatment FEV_1; receiving more bronchodilator treatments or corticosteroids during hospital visits; previous exacerbations (>3 in the past 2 years); previous antibiotic treatment (mainly with ampicillin); and comorbid conditions, such as CHF or coronary artery disease.

Etiology

Although respiratory infections are assumed to be the main risk factors for exacerbation of COPD, other factors are also involved (Table 8-1). Health education for patients, smoking cessation, long-acting bronchodilators (long-acting β-agonists [LABAs] and anticholinergics), inhaled corticosteroids, pulmonary rehabilitation, good nutritional status, and early medical intervention are all considered helpful in preventing exacerbations.

Role of Infection

A variety of microorganisms have been shown to be associated with exacerbations of COPD, including *Haemophilus influenzae*, *Haemophilus parainfluenzae*, *Moraxella catarrhalis*, and *Streptococcus pneumoniae*. A minority of these patients have atypical pathogens such as *Mycoplasma pneumoniae* and *Chlamydia pneumoniae*, but because of limitations regarding diagnosis, the true prevalence of these organisms is not known (see Figure 2-17). Bronchoscopic studies using a sterile, protected specimen brush have shown that 25% of stable patients with stable COPD carry potentially pathogenic bacteria (*H influenzae*, *S pneumoniae*, and *M catarrhalis,* usually <10^3 organisms). During an acute exacerbation of COPD, a much larger percentage of patients (50% to 75%) will demonstrate growth of pathogenic microorganisms in significantly higher concentrations (>10^4 organisms).

Table 8-1: Risk Factors for Acute Exacerbation of COPD

Common

- Environmental conditions
- High air pollution exposure
- Allergic conditions
- Infectious process:
  - Viral: *Rhinovirus* sp, influenza
  - Bacteria: *H influenzae*, *S pneumoniae*, *M catarrhalis*, Enterobacteriaceae, *Pseudomonas* sp

Other

- Inappropriate use of bronchodilator therapy
- No influenza vaccinations
- Use of supplemental oxygen therapy
- Noncompliance with long-term oxygen therapy
- Active or passive smoking
- Occupational exposures
- Nonpulmonary rehabilitation

Several recent studies have demonstrated that patients with the most severe obstructive lung disease have a significantly higher prevalence of gram-negative organisms such as Enterobacteriaceae, and *Pseudomonas* species. Eller et al evaluated sputum cultures from 112 hospital in-patients with acute exacerbations of chronic bronchitis (AECB). Sixty-four percent of patients with a predicted $FEV_1 \leq 35\%$ vs only 30% of those with $FEV_1 \geq 50\%$ (P=0.016) had evidence of gram-negative organisms. The most commonly isolated organisms (from these patients with severe obstructive lung disease) included Entero-bacteriaceae, *Pseudomonas* species, *Proteus vulgaris*, *Serratia marcescens*, *Stenotrophomonas maltophilia*, and *Escherichia coli*.

Miravitlles et al published a study that supported these findings. These investigators evaluated the relationship between FEV_1 and diverse pathogens isolated in the sputum of 91 patients with COPD who presented with type 1 (severe) or type 2 (moderate) symptoms of AECB. Patients were separated into groups by FEV_1 (≥50% vs <50% predicted). There were significantly larger numbers of *H influenzae* and *Pseudomonas aeruginosa* in the group with FEV_1 <50% predicted (*P*<0.05). In contrast, there were significantly larger numbers of benign microorganisms in the group with FEV_1 ≥50% (*P*<0.05). These authors also performed a multivariate analysis with logistic regression and found that *H influenzae* was cultured significantly more commonly in patients who were active smokers (odds ratio [OR] 8.2, confidence interval [CI] 1.9-43) and whose FEV_1 was <50% predicted (OR 6.85, CI 1.6-52). *P aeruginosa* was also cultured significantly more frequently in those with poor lung function, FEV_1<50% (OR 6.6, CI 1.2-124) (Figure 8-4).

The role of bacterial pathogens in AECB is controversial. In some studies, the rates of isolation of bacterial pathogens from sputum were the same during acute exacerbations and stable disease. However, these studies did not differentiate among strains within a bacterial species and therefore could not detect changes in strains over time. Sethi et al hypothesized that the acquisition of a new strain of a pathogenic bacterial species is associated with AECB. These investigators conducted a prospective study in which clinical information and sputum samples for culture were collected monthly and during exacerbations from 81 outpatients with COPD. Molecular typing of sputum isolates of nonencapsulated *H influenzae*, *M catarrhalis*, *S pneumoniae*, and *P aeruginosa* was performed. During

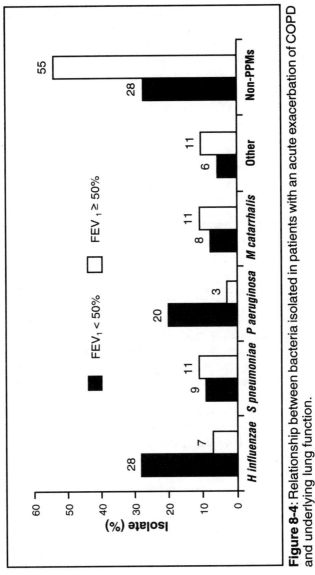

Figure 8-4: Relationship between bacteria isolated in patients with an acute exacerbation of COPD and underlying lung function.

133

56 months, the 81 patients made a total of 1,975 clinic visits, 374 of which occurred during exacerbations (mean, 2.1 per patient per year). On the basis of molecular typing, an exacerbation was diagnosed at 33.0% of the clinic visits that involved isolation of a new strain of bacterial pathogen, as compared with 15.4% of visits at which no new strain was isolated ($P<0.001$; relative risk of an exacerbation, 2.15; 95% CI, 1.83 to 2.53). Isolation of a new strain of *H influenzae*, *M catarrhalis*, or *S pneumoniae* was associated with a significantly increased risk of an exacerbation. Thus the association between an exacerbation and the isolation of a new strain of a bacterial pathogen supports the causative role of bacteria in AECB (Figure 8-5).

Antibiotic Resistance

Until the early 1980s, most bacteria-species-associated AECB could be assumed to be sensitive to ampicillin, erythromycin, tetracycline, and trimethoprim/sulfamethoxazole (TMP/SMX) (Bactrim®, Septra®). These antibiotics were used to manage these exacerbations, but in the 1990s the emergence of bacterial resistance significantly compromised their use. The report from several surveillance studies showed that 35% to 40% of *H influenzae* and 95% to 100% of *M catarrhalis* isolates produced a β-lactamase enzyme. This enzyme induces antibiotic resistance by inactivating antibiotics such as ampicillin and erythromycin. Another important finding of these studies was the identification of several β-lactamase-positive strains of *H influenzae* that showed resistance to amoxicillin/clavulanic acid (Augmentin®). These organisms were also resistant to TMP/SMX and tetracycline up to 50% of the time.

Penicillin-resistant *S pneumoniae* (PRSP) has recently emerged. Before 1992, fewer than 1% of pneumococci in the United States demonstrated high-level resistance. Data from several surveillance studies, including the Centers for Disease Control and Prevention's (CDC) Tracking Resistance in the United States Today (TRUST) that have

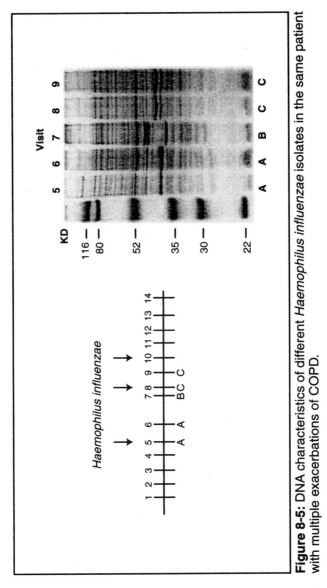

Figure 8-5: DNA characteristics of different *Haemophilus influenzae* isolates in the same patient with multiple exacerbations of COPD.

135

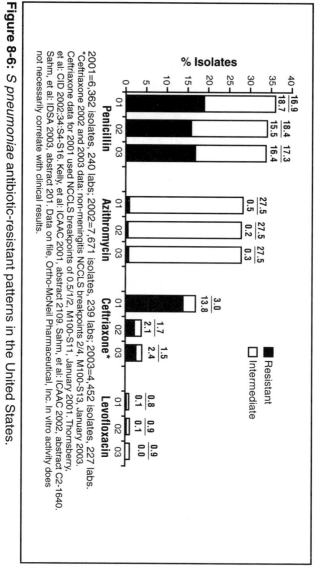

Figure 8-6: *S pneumoniae* antibiotic-resistant patterns in the United States.

2001=6,362 isolates, 240 labs; 2002=7,671 isolates, 239 labs; 2003=4,452 isolates, 227 labs.
*Ceftriaxone 2002 and 2003 data: non-meningitis NCCLS breakpoints 2/4, M100-S13, January 2003.
Ceftriaxone data for 2001 used NCCLS breakpoints of 0.5/1/2, M100-S11, January 2001. Thornsberry, et al: CID 2002;34:S4-S16. Kelly, et al: ICAAC 2001, abstract 2109. Sahm, et al: ICAAC 2002, abstract C2-1640. Sahm, et al: IDSA 2003, abstract 201. Data on file, Ortho-McNeil Pharmaceutical, Inc. In vitro activity does not necessarily correlate with clinical results.

collected information since 1995 have shown that in 2003 up to 35% of isolates were PRSP; 24% were intermediately susceptible, and 10% to 15% were highly resistant (Figure 8-6). PRSP resistance is classified as high if the minimal inhibitory concentration (MIC) is more than 2 mg/mL. PRSP isolates are also known to be associated with decreased susceptibility to other antibiotics including cephalosporins (clindamycin [Cleocin®], lincomycin [Lincocin®]), macrolides (Biaxin®, Zithromax®), TMP/SMX, and tetracyclines. The resistance rates to macrolides are comparable for clarithromycin, erythromycin, and azithromycin. A study conducted in the winter of 1993 to 1994 found that the resistance of *S pneumoniae* to macrolides was 20%, but by 1996 to 1997 and up to 2003, the resistance was reported as 30% to 40%. Later studies have also reported PRSP isolates resistant to cefuroxime (100%, Ceftin®, Zinacef®), amoxicillin/clavulanate (94%, Augmentin®), and cefotaxime (73%, Claforan®). In the United States, PRSP is not associated with decreased susceptibility to quinolones. Most fluoroquinolones (levofloxacin [Levaquin®], gatifloxacin [Tequin®], moxifloxacin [Avelox®], and gemifloxacin [Factive®]) exhibit enhanced activity against *S pneumoniae*. The PRSP isolates are also susceptible to these antibiotics.

Clinical studies have identified risk factors that are present in patients who have PRSP infections (Table 8-2). These modifying factors have to be considered when choosing antibiotics to treat patients with AECB.

Evaluation
Clinical
Listed below are the key components of the history, physical examination, and laboratory evaluation a physician should obtain during evaluation of an acute exacerbation of COPD. The formulation of therapy and the criteria for the choice of ambulatory treatment or hospital admission are listed as well.

Table 8-2: Clinical Risk Factors Associated With Penicillin-Resistant and Multidrug-Resistant *Streptococccus Pneumoniae**

- Age >65 years
- β-lactam and macrolide therapy within 3 months
- Alcoholism
- Immune suppression (including use of corticosteroids)
- Multiple medical comorbidities
- Exposure to child in daycare

*These factors have been identified in patients with community-acquired pneumonia. Modified from Niederman et al: *Am J Resp Crit Care Med* 2001;163:1730-1754.

History
- Duration and progression of symptoms
- Sputum volume and other characteristics
- Dyspnea—severity
- Baseline respiratory conditions—pulmonary function tests
- History of previous exacerbation or hospitalization within the last year
- Comorbidities—acute or chronic
- Exercise limitations
- Sleep and eating difficulties
- Home therapeutic regimens
- Influenza vaccination history
- Health-care resources use

Physical Examination

- Hemodynamic instability (ie, heart rate, arterial blood pressure)
- Respiratory rate
- Altered mental status
- Use of accessory muscles (paroxysmal abdominal retractions/use of accessory respiratory muscles)
- Wheezes
- Findings of acute comorbid conditions (ie, cor pulmonale, pneumonia).

Laboratory Testing

This testing is mainly recommended for patients who will require hospitalization.

Blood tests: White blood cell counts; biochemistry evaluation/electrolytes; renal and liver function serum drug concentrations.

Microbiology: Sputum Gram stain and culture; serology—atypical organisms.

Assessment of oxygenation: Pulse oximetry monitoring; arterial blood gases.

Chest Radiographs

For patients who require treatment in the emergency department or hospital admission, chest radiographs are useful diagnostic tests. Several cohort studies have found abnormalities in 16% to 21% of patients that prompted a change in management. Most of the patients had new pulmonary infiltrates or evidence of CHF. Therefore, we recommend that in patients with acute exacerbation, a chest radiograph be obtained to rule out any other abnormalities.

Spirometry

Observational studies have shown that a spirometric assessment at presentation or during treatment of acute exacerbation of COPD is not useful in judging the severity of the illness or guiding the management of the patient. When measured at the time of exacerbation, FEV_1 showed no significant correlation with

Table 8-3: Pharmacotherapy for Acute Exacerbations of Chronic Lung Disease

Bronchodilator therapy	Short-acting β_2-agonists, by MDI with spacer
Corticosteroids	Oral prednisone therapy, 40 mg PO qd, for 7-10 days
Theophylline	Due to poor safety profile, its use is not recommended.

PO_2 and only weak correlation with PCO_2. A study by Emmerman et al in 199 patients who presented to the emergency department with acute exacerbation of COPD demonstrated that peak expiratory flow rate (PEFR) and FEV_1 are correlated ($r=0.84$; $P<0.001$). The clinical implications of these findings, however, are unclear. Furthermore, in this study, a substantial minority of patients had absolute discrepancy with this percentage-predicted FEV_1 and percentage-predicted PEFR >10 points. At present, no data support the routine use of peak flow meters or FEV_1 assessment to manage COPD exacerbations and therefore, we do not recommend it.

Other

• Electrocardiogram: only in the emergency department.

The objectives of pharmacotherapy during an acute exacerbation of COPD were summarized in the ATS/ERS consensus statement and include: improve the patient's symptoms; treat underlying infection if present; avoid additional invasive therapeutic maneuvers; increase the length of time between exacerbations (exacerbation-free interval); provide treatment as an outpatient; and decrease the need for hospitalization.

Ipratropium bromide, MDI alone or in
combination with short-acting β_2-agonist

If the patient cannot tolerate PO therapy, short
course of IV methylprednisolone.

MDI = metered-dose inhaler

Bronchodilator Therapy

The bronchodilators used to treat acute exacerbations
of COPD are short-acting β_2-agonists, LABAs, and anticholinergic agents (Table 8-3). Limited clinical data suggest that formoterol (a long-acting β-agonist, [Foradil®,
Symbicort®]) can be used during an acute exacerbation
of COPD.

The clinical studies available have shown that short-
acting β_2-agonists and ipratropium bromide (Atrovent®,
Combivent®) are equally efficacious during acute exacerbations. While some studies suggest that adding ipratropium
bromide to a short- or long-acting β_2-agonist improves the
patient's spirometry and clinical response, other studies
do not. The current clinical practice is to first use a short-
acting β_2-agonist and then add ipratropium bromide if the
patient's symptoms do not improve. These agents may be
used concomitantly.

The inhaled route for delivering these drugs has been
shown to result in fewer adverse events and maximum efficacy. Patients can receive metered-dose inhalers (MDIs)
in combination with devices such as large-volume attachments (spacers), breath-attenuated MDIs, and dry-powder

inhalers. The techniques for using MDIs and their attachments must be taught to the patients and reinforced. Drug deposition may vary among delivery systems. Nebulization has been a preferred delivery mode during acute exacerbations mainly because patients may have difficulty in using MDI devices. The safety and value of continued drug nebulization delivery have not been established in COPD. Randomized controlled trials using MDI vs nebulization have not shown the superiority of continuous nebulization therapy. In mechanically ventilated patients, bronchodilator delivery via MDI with a spacer has a higher particle deposition as compared to a nebulizer. The dose schedule for β_2-agonists and ipratropium bromide during an acute exacerbation has not been established.

There is no evidence that oral or intravenous β_2-agonists improve bronchodilator response. Therefore, these routes of administration are not recommended. High doses of β_2-agonists are known to be associated with increased side effects, including tachyarrhythmias, tremor, and morbidity. Recent studies have described the increased rate of cardiac events associated with β_2-agonists in patients with COPD and failed to show a benefit of regular use of albuterol (Proventil® HFA, Ventolin® HFA) in stable patients. Short-acting β_2-agonists may be associated with an idiosyncratic bronchoconstriction response and tachyphylaxis with a decrease in the patient's clinical response.

Ipratropium bromide has been demonstrated to have minimal side effects, primarily unpleasant taste and cough. There is no evidence that patients on ipratropium bromide can develop a tolerance to chronic therapy.

Methylxanthines:
Theophylline and/or Aminophylline

Theophylline (Slo-Bid®, Theo-Dur®) and theophylline/aminophylline (Primatene® Dual Action®) have been shown to have comparable or less bronchodilator effect than β_2-agonists or anticholinergic agents. The major limitation of these drugs is the need for continuous blood-level monitoring, and their side effects include cardiac arrhythmias, electrolyte imbalances, and extensive drug interactions. Because of these issues, we do not recommend the use of methylxanthines in the treatment of acute exacerbations.

Treatment With Corticosteroids

Corticosteroids are recommended in most cases of acute exacerbation of COPD. There is a consensus that patients with significant bronchodilator response are more likely to benefit from this therapy, but the reason is not well established. Corticosteroids can be administered intravenously, orally, and by inhalation. Limited data exist on the use of inhaled corticosteroids during an acute exacerbation of COPD.

Albert et al published the first randomized, double-blind, placebo-controlled trial of systemic corticosteroids in the treatment of acute exacerbation of COPD. A regimen of IV methylprednisolone (Medrol®) q.i.d. for 3 days produced an early improvement in FEV_1 that was observed during the treatment period. Recent studies have suggested that a short course of oral prednisone (Deltasone®, Liquid Pred®) therapy can be useful. A 2-week course of 30 mg daily oral prednisone in patients with severe airflow obstruction resulted in a significantly lower rate of treatment failure, a decreased length of hospital stay, and a more rapid improvement in FEV_1. In the largest study published to date, the Systemic Corticosteroids in Chronic Obstructive Pulmonary Disease Exacerbations (SCCOPE) study, 271 patients with an acute exacerbation of COPD received placebo or a two-dose regimen of corticosteroid therapy for 2 or 8 weeks. For the combined glucocorticoid group, the risk for treatment failure as compared to placebo was reduced by 10 percentage points (33% vs 23%, respectively), and FEV_1 improved statistically significantly during the first 3 days of therapy. There was no difference in FEV_1 after 2 weeks. The SC-

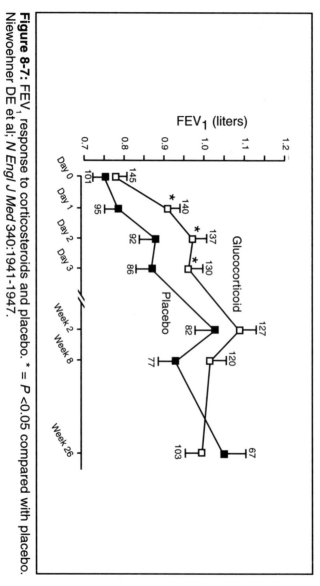

Figure 8-7: FEV$_1$ response to corticosteroids and placebo. * = P <0.05 compared with placebo. Niewoehner DE et al; *N Engl J Med* 340:1941-1947.

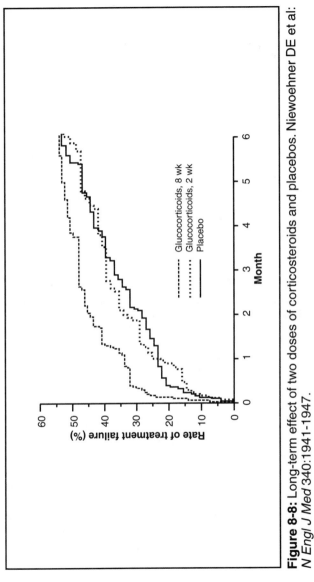

Figure 8-8: Long-term effect of two doses of corticosteroids and placebos. Niewoehner DE et al: *N Engl J Med* 340:1941-1947.

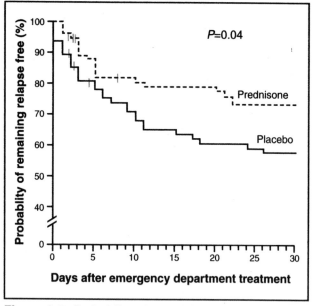

Figure 8-9: Probability of remaining relapse free after treatment with oral prednisone 40 mg daily or placebo in patients with acute exacerbation of COPD.

COPE trial demonstrated equivalent outcome between 2-week and 8-week corticosteroid regimens (Figures 8-7 and 8-8).

Recent studies have suggested that a short course of oral prednisone therapy can be useful. A 2-week course of 30 mg to 40 mg daily oral prednisone in patients with severe airflow obstruction resulted in significantly lower rates of treatment failure, decreased lengths of hospital stay, and more rapid improvement in FEV_1 (Figure 8-9). Because all the published studies have excluded patients who received systemic corticosteroids within the preceding month, it is not known if corticosteroid treatment is also efficacious in these patients.

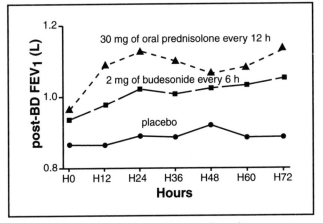

Figure 8-10: Comparison of lung function response (FEV$_1$) in patients treated with nebulized budesonide, prednisolone, or placebo.

Inhaled nebulized corticosteroids (budesonide [Pulmicort®, Rhinocort®]) also improve post-bronchodilator FEV$_1$ and can be safely used in patients with acute exacerbation of COPD (Figure 8-10). Regular use of inhaled corticosteroids may reduce the numbers of annual exacerbations. The appropriate duration of therapy is 5 days to 2 weeks. The 10-day course has been studied the most thoroughly.

Well-known side effects of systemic corticosteroids are the major limiting factors of this therapy. The SCCOPE trial showed that hyperglycemia was significantly more common in patients who received corticosteroids compared with placebo. In patients with COPD, corticosteroid-induced myopathy may be more common than was initially appreciated. Histologically, both myopathic changes and generalized muscle fiber atrophy have been reported. In one study, survival of patients with steroid-induced myopathy was significantly lower compared to those without myopathy but with similar airflow obstruction.

Treatment With Antibiotics

The specific etiology of acute exacerbation of COPD is difficult to determine in an outpatient office setting on the basis of symptoms and signs. Sputum studies, although potentially useful, have significant limitations of delay in obtaining results, cost, and lack of sensitivity and specificity. Recent treatment guidelines for acute exacerbation of COPD reflect the lack of evidence-based data to provide specific recommendations for the use of antibiotics. The Global Initiative for Chronic Obstructive Lung Disease (GOLD) guideline, which was a National Heart, Lung and Blood Institute/World Health Organization (NHLBI/WHO) initiative for COPD recommends that antibiotic choices be made on the basis of local sensitivity patterns of the most common pathogens associated with acute exacerbation of COPD.

A number of clinical trials examined the use of antibiotics to treat acute exacerbation of COPD. Many of the earlier studies showed either no benefit or minimal benefit from antibiotics. Some of the more recent publications, including a meta-analysis, demonstrated a benefit of antibiotics during an acute exacerbation, but not for preventing them. In 1987, Anthonisen et al reported the results of a large-scale placebo-controlled trial designed to determine the effectiveness of antibiotics in treating acute exacerbation of COPD. In this study, 173 patients with chronic bronchitis were followed for 3.5 years, during which they had 362 exacerbations. This study finally brought some conformity to the definition of acute exacerbation of COPD and was the first widely accepted classification for the severity of presenting symptoms. Patients who were classified in the severe range of acute exacerbation of COPD included those with all three clinical symptoms (increased shortness of breath, increased sputum production, and a change in sputum purulence) at initial presentation. The patients were randomized to antibiotics or placebo in a double-blind, crossover fashion. Three oral antibiotics chosen by the physician were used for 10 days: amoxicillin, TMP/SMX, and doxycycline. Approximately 40% of all exacerbations were type 1 (severe), 40% were type 2 (moderate), and only 20% were type 3 (mild). Patients with the most severe exacerbations (type 1) received a significant benefit from antibiotics, whereas there was no significant difference between antibiotic and placebo in patients who had only one of the defined symptoms (type 3). Overall, the antibiotic-treated patients showed a more rapid improvement in peak flow, a greater percentage of clinical success, and a smaller percentage of clinical failure than those who received placebo. In addition, the period of illness was 2 days shorter for the antibiotic-treated group. The major criticisms of this study were that no microbiology tests were performed and that all antibiotics were assumed to be equivalent.

Allegra et al found significant benefit to the use of amoxicillin/clavulanate acid therapy compared with placebo for patients with severe disease. Patients who received this antibiotic exhibited a higher success rate (86.4% vs 50.3% in the placebo group, $P<0.01$) and a lower frequency of recurrent exacerbations. In 1995, Saint et al published the results of a meta-analysis examining the role of antibiotics in the treatment of acute exacerbation of COPD (Figure 8-11). These investigators analyzed nine randomized, placebo-controlled trials published between 1957 and 1992. Unfortunately, no common outcome reported in each of the studies was included in this analysis. However, some outcomes available for analysis and comparison in many of the studies include: (1) the mean number of days of illness, (2) the overall symptom score, and (3) the changes in PEFR. Using this form of analysis, the antibiotic-treated patients showed an overall, statistically significant benefit. Analysis of the studies that provided data on expiratory flow rates found an improvement of 10.75 L/min in this group. The authors concluded that this antibiotic-associ-

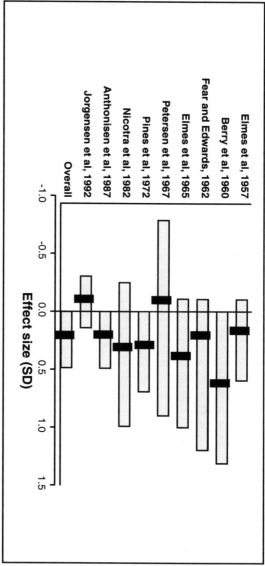

Figure 8-11: Effect sizes (mean differences in outcome divided by the pooled standard deviation) in nine studies on the use of antibiotics for exacerbations of COPD. Horizontal lines denote 95% confidence intervals. The data indicate a significant improvement due to antibiotic therapy.

ated improvement is likely to be clinically significant, particularly for patients with low baseline peak flow rates and limited respiratory reserve.

There are additional potential benefits to antibiotic therapy for patients with acute exacerbation of COPD. Antibiotics can reduce the burden of bacteria in the airway. Bronchoscopic studies using a sterile protected specimen brush have demonstrated that 25% of stable COPD patients are colonized (usually $<10^3$ organisms) with potentially pathogenic bacteria. However, a much larger percentage (50% to 75%) of patients with acute exacerbations carry potentially pathogenic microorganisms in addition to significantly higher concentrations (frequently $>10^4$ organisms) of bacteria in the large airways. Because treatment with appropriate antibiotics significantly decreases the bacterial burden (and frequently eradicates the sensitive organisms) at the 72-hour follow-up bronchoscopy, it is speculated that the proper choice of antibiotic reduces the risk of progression to more severe infections, such as pneumonia. The eradication of bacteria by antibiotics is thought to break the vicious cycle of infection, ie, lung destruction leading to progression of the lung disease.

Another study, by Novira et al, recently reported similar findings of gram-negative pathogens in a prospective, randomized, double-blind, placebo-controlled trial evaluating the use of ofloxacin (Floxin®) in 90 consecutive patients with acute exacerbation of COPD who required mechanical ventilation. This study demonstrated a significant number of gram-negative organisms (including *E coli*, *Proteus mirabilis*, and *P aeruginosa*) in the patients with severe acute exacerbation of COPD. In addition to supporting the findings of the previously reported studies, this trial demonstrated that eradicating these pathogens is important for improving outcomes in this high-risk population. The antibiotic-treated group had a significantly lower in-hospital mortality rate (4% vs 22%, $P=0.01$) and a significantly reduced length of stay in the hospital (14.9 vs 24.5, $P=0.01$)

compared with the placebo group. In addition, the patients receiving ofloxacin were less likely to develop pneumonia than those on placebo, especially during the first week of mechanical ventilation (mean ± standard deviation: 7.2±2.2 days [range 4-11] vs 10.6±2.9 days [range 9-14], $P=0.04$ by log-rank test).

If the use of antibiotics to treat acute exacerbation of COPD has all the potential benefits discussed, does it matter which agent is chosen? The Anthonisen et al study assumed that all of the antibiotics were equivalent; thus, the specific agent prescribed was not considered important. Moreover, most of the recently published antibiotic trials were designed to compare a new antibiotic with an established compound for the purpose of registration and licensing. Equivalence is the desired outcome of such trials and therefore the agent chosen for comparison is not considered important. In addition, these trials frequently include patients with poorly defined disease severity (often without any obstructive lung disease) and acute illness of minor severity.

Another problem with interpreting the literature on acute exacerbation of COPD is the great variation in time frame (48 hours to 28 days) that is used to assess patients for relapse or resolution of symptoms. Relapse can most clearly be defined as treatment failure resulting in a return doctor visit due to persistent or worsening symptoms. However, many patients do not seek medical care, despite persistent symptoms. The published relapse rates for patients with acute exacerbation of COPD range from 17% to 32%. Despite the problems with many of the published antibiotic trials, some retrospective trials emphasize the importance of choosing the correct antibiotic for treatment of patients with acute exacerbation of COPD.

A recent retrospective study of outpatients with documented COPD, conducted at our institution, evaluated the risk factors for therapy failure 14 days after an acute exacerbation. The participating patients had 362 exacerbations during 18 months. One group received antibiotics (270 visits) and the second group (92 visits) did not. Both groups had similar demographics and severity of underlying COPD. The patients' mean age was 67 ± 10 years ($\pm$ SD), 100% of patients had >50 pack-per-year smoking history, and 45% were active smokers. Based on the American Thoracic Society's COPD classification, 39% had mild disease, 47% had moderate disease, and 14% had severe disease. Most patients (95%) with severe symptoms at presentation (Type 1) received antibiotics, vs only 40% with mild symptoms. The overall relapse rate (defined as a return visit with persistent or worsening symptoms within 14 days) was 22%. After an extensive multivariate analysis, the major risk factor for relapse was lack of antibiotic therapy (32% vs 19%, $P<0.001$ compared to the antibiotic-treated group).

The type of antibiotic used was also an important variable associated with the 14-day treatment failure. Patients treated with amoxicillin had a 54% relapse rate compared with only 13% for the other antibiotics ($P<0.01$). Furthermore, treatment with amoxicillin resulted in a higher incidence of failure, even when compared with those who did not receive antibiotics ($P=0.006$) (Figure 8-6). Other variables, such as COPD severity, types of exacerbation, prior or concomitant use of corticosteroids, and current use of chronic oxygen therapy were not significantly associated with the 14-day relapse. This study showed that the use of antibiotics was associated with a significantly lower rate of therapy failure.

In contrast to Anthonisen's data, our data show that antibiotics are beneficial regardless of the severity of acute exacerbation of COPD (ie, those with mild acute exacerbation of COPD still gained benefit from treatment with antibiotics). Furthermore, the patients who received antibiotics and failed within 14 days had a significantly higher rate of hospital admissions than those who did not receive antibiotics. Although there may be many explanations for these treatment failures, the most likely one is that the pathogens were resistant to amoxicillin.

Destache et al reported the impact of antibiotic selection, antimicrobial efficacy, and related cost in acute exacerbation of COPD. This study was a retrospective review of 60 outpatients from the pulmonary clinic of a teaching institution who were diagnosed with COPD and chronic bronchitis. The participating patients had a total of 224 episodes of acute exacerbation of COPD requiring antibiotic treatment. The antibiotics were arbitrarily divided into three groups: first-line (amoxicillin, cotrimoxazole, erythromycin, and tetracycline); second-line (cephradine [Anspor®, Velosef®], cefuroxime [Kefurox®, Zinacef®], cefaclor [Ceclor®], cefprozil [Cefzil®]); and third-line (amoxicillin/clavulanate, azithromycin, and ciprofloxacin [Cipro®]) agents. The failure rates were significantly higher (at 14 days) for the first-line agents compared with the third-line agents (19% vs 7%, $P<0.05$). When compared with those who received the first-line agents, the patients treated with the third-line agents had a significantly longer time between exacerbations (34 weeks vs 17 weeks, $P<0.02$), overall fewer hospitalizations (3/26 [12%] vs 18/26 [69%] patients, $P<0.02$), and considerably lower total cost ($542 vs $942, $P<0.0001$).

Based on the results of these studies, in addition to widespread reports of increasing antimicrobial resistance to the common pathogens isolated in patients with acute exacerbation of COPD, appropriate antibiotic selection is extremely important. Therefore, it is not only essential to treat these patients with antibiotics, it is critical to choose the appropriate ones.

End Point for the Treatment of Acute Exacerbation of COPD

Conventional end points for efficacy of antibiotic treatment in acute exacerbation of COPD include the symptoms and bacteriologic resolution measured at 2 to

3 weeks after the treatment was started. Most of these end points rely solely on the subjective report of symptoms' improvement. These end points have been used for drug registration purposes but lack clinical relevance. It has been suggested by several reports that the infection-free interval, ie, the time to the next episode of acute exacerbation of COPD, may be a more suitable end point in this patient population.

According to Wilson et al, patients with acute exacerbation of COPD treated with gemifloxacin showed a significant increase in the infection-free interval as compared with clarithromycin. This end point may reflect the ability of the antibiotic to achieve adequate bacteriologic eradication in the airway. This study showed that this end point was associated with decreased hospitalization rates. This can now be translated into cost savings, improved quality of life, and potentially slower progression of the underlying airway obstruction.

Clinical Parameters to Stratify Patients Into Risk Groups

Because the morbidity and mortality of acute exacerbation of COPD are high, many investigators have attempted to describe characteristics that could be used to stratify the patients into risk groups. Some studies have validated a few of the following risk factors for treatment failure, while others show different factors associated with increased risk of relapse. Despite these conflicting studies, the clinical parameters that are implicated as possible risk factors for treatment failure in acute exacerbation of COPD include: (1) older age (>65 years old), (2) severe underlying COPD (FEV_1 <35% predicted), (3) frequent exacerbations (≥4/year), (4) more severe symptoms at presentation (Anthonisen et al types: 1 [severe] and 2 [moderate]), (5) comorbidities (especially cardiopulmonary disease, but also CHF, diabetes mellitus, chronic renal failure, and chronic liver disease), and (6) prolonged history of COPD (>10 years). Some authors state that many infections in acute exacerbation of COPD are noninvasive and will eventually resolve spontaneously. However, because the costs of failed treatment remain high, better strategies are needed for the treatment of these exacerbations.

Niederman et al recently reported that age >65 years and inpatient treatment are the major determinants contributing to the overall cost of acute exacerbation of COPD. The cost was estimated at $1.2 billion for the 207,540 in-patients ≥65 years old vs only $452 million for 5.8 million outpatients in the same age group. The mean length of stay was longer, and the in-hospital mortality rate was significantly higher for those >65 years of age.

Based on the concept of risk stratification of patients by clinical parameters, a target approach for the treatment of acute exacerbation of COPD has been proposed by the Canadian Respiratory Society and the ATS/ERS statement. This group developed a classification for patients presenting with symptoms of acute bronchitis using the following factors: (1) number and severity of acute symptoms, (2) age, (3) severity of airflow obstruction (measured by FEV_1), (4) frequency of exacerbations, and (5) history of comorbid conditions. This symposium suggested that patients could be adequately profiled into different categories. Acute bronchitis (Group 1) includes healthy people without previous respiratory problems. 'Simple' acute exacerbation of COPD (Group 2) includes those patients whose age is <65 years, those who have had ≤4 exacerbations per year, those with minimal or no impairment in lung function (by pulmonary function tests), and those without any comorbid conditions. 'Complicated' acute exacerbation of COPD (Group 3) includes patients older than 65 years, those with FEV_1 <50% predicted, or those with ≥4 exacerbations per year. Finally, 'complicated' acute exacerbation of COPD with associated comorbid illnesses (Group 4) includes patients with CHF, liver disease, diabetes, or chronic renal failure (Table 8-4).

Table 8-4: Patient Profiles From the Canadian Chronic Bronchitis Guidelines

Acute Bronchitis (Group 1)

- Healthy people without previous respiratory problems

'Simple' Chronic Bronchitis (Group 2)

- Age ≤65 years old *and*
- ≤4 exacerbations per year *and*
- Minimal or no impairment in pulmonary function *and*
- No comorbid conditions

'Complicated' Chronic Bronchitis (Group 3)

- Age >65 years old *or*
- FEV_1 <50% predicted *or*
- ≥4 exacerbations per year

'Complicated' Chronic Bronchitis With Comorbid Illness (Group 4)

Above criteria for Group 3, *plus*:

- Congestive heart failure *or*
- Diabetes *or*
- Chronic renal failure *or*
- Chronic liver disease *or*
- Other chronic disease

Adapted from Balter MS, et al: Canadian guidelines for the management of acute exacerbations of chronic bronchitis. *Can Respir J* 2003;10(suppl B):3B-32B.

The 'Ideal' Antibiotic for the Treatment of Acute Exacerbation of COPD

Characteristics of the ideal antibiotics to be considered when choosing these agents for patients with acute exacerbation of COPD include:

1. Significant activity against the most common pathogens isolated in patients with acute exacerbation of COPD and whether there are substantial gaps in the coverage of these organisms.

2. Adequate coverage of the most likely pathogens in patients with acute exacerbations of COPD based on patient profiles that define the most likely spectrum of etiologic pathogens. As previously described, this is especially important in patients with severe underlying obstructive lung disease, who are more commonly infected with gram-negative organisms than those with mild COPD. Additionally, patients with risk factors for a more complicated course (those in Group 3 [Complicated] and Group 4 [Complicated with comorbid conditions]) should be prescribed antibiotics with adequate coverage for the usual pathogens in acute exacerbation of COPD, as well as for gram-negative organisms.

3. Susceptibility of the antimicrobial agent to the likely pathogens in acute exacerbation of COPD. There is an increasing prevalence of *H influenzae and M catarrhalis* that produce bacterial enzymes, which inactivate traditional β-lactam antibiotics. Additionally, a growing number of these organisms are resistant to many of the antibiotics that are now available. It is important to know which of the mechanisms of resistance of these agents are clinically important for the treatment of acute exacerbation of COPD. It is also critical to know the local resistance rates of these microorganisms before prescribing a specific antibiotic for therapy. Chapter 2 examines the resistance of these organisms to many of the antibiotics that are commonly used to treat acute exacerbation of COPD.

4. Good penetration into sputum, bronchial mucosa, and epithelial lining. The goal of antimicrobial therapy is to deliver the appropriate drug to the specific site of infection. In acute exacerbation of COPD, the bacteria are predominantly found in the airway lumens, along the mucosal cell surfaces, and within the mucosal tissue. Various antibiotic classes exhibit markedly different degrees of penetration into the tissues and secretions of the respiratory tract. Although no studies demonstrate that the concentration of antibiotics at one particular intrapulmonary site is better than at any other site, the concentrations of antibiotics in sputum, bronchial mucosa, epithelial lining fluid, and macrophages are thought to be predictive of clinical efficacy. These antibiotics exhibit a concentration-effect relationship.

5. Easy to take with minimal side effects. In a recent survey, patient compliance was demonstrated to be significantly improved when medications were given once or twice a day, rather than three or more times a day. Additionally, shorter courses of therapy (5 to 7 days) were associated with better compliance. Of the patients interviewed, >80% stated a preference for once or twice daily dosing, and >54% admitted to noncompliance with the prescribed regimen (taking the antibiotic sporadically or not completing the full course).

6. Cost-effective, considering more than acquisition cost of antibiotics. Clearly multiple factors should be considered when selecting an antibiotic for the treatment of acute exacerbation of COPD, in addition to just the acquisition cost. These other economic end points are important when defining the cost-effectiveness of any particular antibiotic, such as: (1) the cost of treatment failures (including the need for further antibiotics and the days of lost work), (2) the amount saved by preventing hospitalization, (3) the duration of disease-free intervals, and (4) the development of antimicrobial resistance. Although there are no adequate cost-effectiveness

data now available to support the use of any particular antibiotic, the importance of these factors is supported by the retrospective studies (previously examined) by Destache et al and Niederman et al.

Hospitalization Criteria

Indications for hospitalization for patients with COPD exacerbation that were recommended by the ATS/ERS statement can be summarized as follows: patients with high-risk comorbid conditions including pulmonary (eg, pneumonia) or nonpulmonary conditions (eg, cor pulmonale, cardiac arrhythmia, CHF); patients with acute exacerbations characterized by increased dyspnea, cough, and sputum production plus one of the following conditions: inadequate response of symptoms to outpatient management; marked increase in dyspnea on exertion; inability to eat or sleep because of dyspnea; worsening hypoxemia; worsening hypercapnia; and/or inability of the patient to care for herself/himself.

Criteria for ICU Admission

Consider ICU or special respiratory care unit admission of patients with acute exacerbation of COPD with one or more of the following:
- Severe dyspnea that has not responded to initial emergency therapy
- Change in patient's mental status
- Evidence of respiratory muscle fatigue, characterized by paroxysmal abdominal motion and/or use of accessory respiratory muscles
- Persistent worsening of hypoxemia despite supplemental oxygen
- Severe worsening of respiratory acidosis (pH <7.25).
- Ventilation, either noninvasive or invasive that cannot be administered in non-ICU setting
- The presence of other end-organ dysfunction, ie, shock, renal, liver, or neurologic disturbance.

Mechanical Ventilation

Mechanical ventilation (MV), either conventional or noninvasive, is not a therapy but a form of life support used until the cause underlying the acute respiratory failure is reversed with medical therapy. Mechanical ventilation should be considered when, despite 'optimal' medical therapy and oxygen administration, one of the following persists: moderate-to-severe dyspnea with evident use of accessory muscles and abdominal paradox; moderate-to-severe acidosis (pH <7.36); and hypercapnia (arterial carbon dioxide tension ($PaCO_2$) >6 to 8 kPa (45 to 60 mm Hg); and/or respiratory frequency >24 breaths/min.

Noninvasive positive pressure ventilation (NPPV) should be offered to patients with exacerbations when respiratory acidosis (pH <7.36) persists after optimal medical therapy and oxygenation (Figure 8-12). If pH <7.30, NPPV should be delivered under controlled environments, such as intermediate ICU and/or high-dependency units. If pH <7.25, NPPV should be administered in the ICU and intubation should be readily available. Contraindications and complications of NPPV are summarized in Table 8-5.

Endotracheal intubation should be considered in patients with the following:

- NPPV failure (worsening of arterial blood gases and/or pH in 1 to 2 h or lack of improvement in arterial blood gases and/or pH after 4 h)
- severe acidosis (pH <7.25) and hypercapnia ($PaCO_2$ >8 kPa (60 mm Hg))
- life-threatening hypoxemia (arterial oxygen tension/inspiratory oxygen fraction <26.6 kPa (200 mm Hg))
- tachypnea >35 breaths/min
- other complications including metabolic abnormalities, sepsis, pneumonia, pulmonary embolism, barotraumas, and massive pleural effusion.

A summary of the treatment recommendations for patients with an acute exacerbation of COPD is shown in Table 8-6.

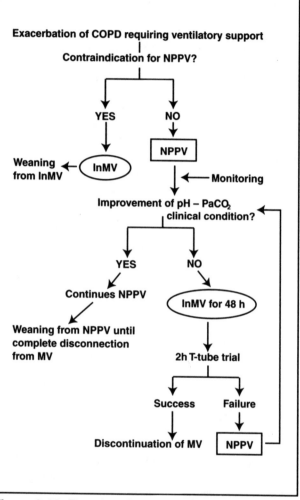

Figure 8-12: Flowchart for the use of NPPV in patients with exacerbation of COPD complicated by acute respiratory failure.

Table 8-5: Contraindications and Complications of NPPV

Contraindications for NPPV include the following:

- Respiratory arrest
- Cardiovascular instability (hypotension, arrhythmias, myocardial infarction)
- Impaired mental status, somnolence, inability to cooperate
- Copious and/or viscous secretions with high aspiration risk
- Recent facial or gastroesophageal surgery
- Craniofacial trauma and/or fixed nasopharyngeal abnormality
- Burns
- Extreme obesity

Complications of NPPV include the following:

- Facial skin erythema
- Nasal congestion
- Nasal bridge ulceration
- Sinus/ear pain
- Nasal/oral dryness
- Eye irritation
- Gastric irritation
- Aspiration pneumonia
- Poor control of secretions

Adapted from Celli BR, MacNee W, ATS/ERS Task Force: Standards for the diagnosis and treatment of patients with COPD: a summary of the ATS/ERS position paper. *Eur Respir J* 2004;23:932-946.

Table 8-6: Summary of Treatment of Acute Exacerbation of COPD

Ambulatory Patients

Treatment

Patient education
- Inhalation techniques
- Use of spacers

Bronchodilators
- Albuterol and ipratropium MDI with spacer, 2 puffs q 4-6 h
- Consider adding long-acting β-agonist if patient is not using one

Corticosteroids
- Prednisone 20 mg PO q.d. for 5 days
- Consider adding inhaled corticosteroids

Antibiotics (based on local bacteria resistance patterns)
- Macrolides (azithromycin, clarithromycin, dirithromycin)
- New cephalosporins (cefpodoxime, cefprozil)
- Doxycycline
- Amoxicillin/ampicillin (depending on local prevalence of bacterial β-lactamases)
- If the patient has taken antibiotics, consider the following:
  - Fluoroquinolones (levofloxacin, gatifloxacin, moxifloxacin) *or*
  - amoxicillin/clavulanate

Hospitalized Patients

Treatment

Bronchodilators
- Albuterol and ipratropium MDI with spacer, 2 puffs q 2-4 h
- Consider adding long-acting β-agonist if patient is not using one

Supplemental oxygen (link to oxygen section)
- Venturi mask—goal oxygen saturation >92 %

Corticosteroids
- If patient tolerates PO—prednisone 20 mg PO q.d. for 5 days
- If patient cannot tolerate PO, methylprednisolone 125 mg every 6 hr for up to 72 hr followed by prednisone 30 mg PO for a total of 14 days
- Consider adding inhaled corticosteroids

Antibiotics (based on local bacteria resistance patterns)
- Fluoroquinolones (levofloxacin, gatifloxacin, moxifloxacin) *or*
- amoxicillin/clavulanate *or*
- macrolides (azithromycin, clarithromycin, dirithromycin)
- If *Pseudomonas* sp is isolated—ciprofloxacin

Adapted from Celli BR, MacNee W, ATS/ERS Task Force: Standards for the diagnosis and treatment of patients with COPD: a summary of the ATS/ERS position paper. *Eur Respir J* 2004;23:932-946.

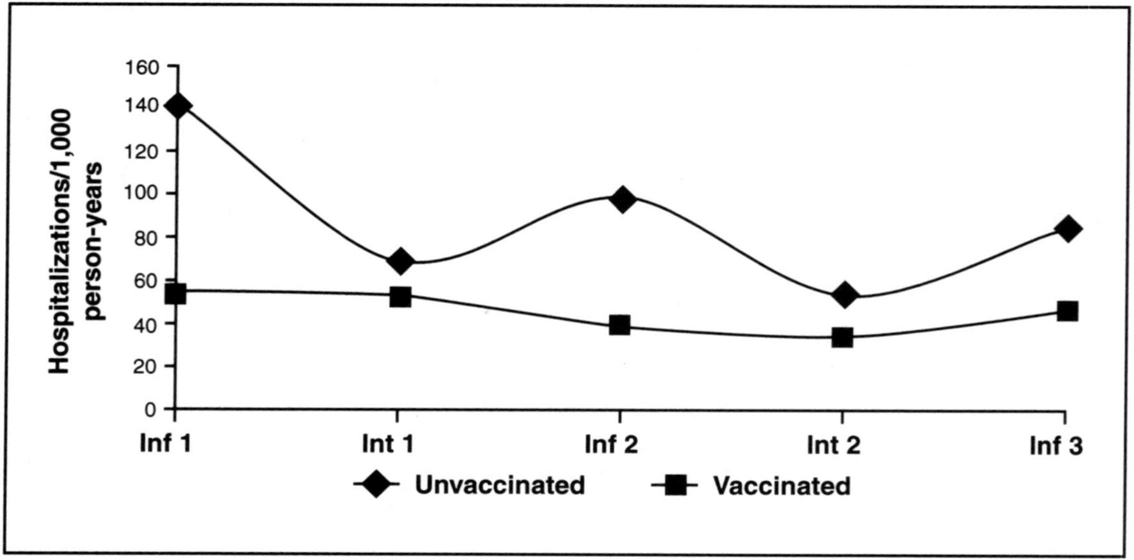

Figure 8-13: Observed annualized rates of hospitalization for pneumonia and influenza among vaccinated and unvaccinated people for each study period.

Prevention

The two most important prevention measures are smoking cessation and active immunizations, including influenza and pneumococcal vaccinations. Smoking cessation is examined in Chapter 5.

Influenza is an important cause of lower respiratory tract infections. Influenza A and B often reach epidemic proportions during the winter months. The impact of influenza is critical to the development of other lower respiratory infections including acute exacerbation of COPD and pneumonia. Epidemiologic studies have shown that the frequency of lower respiratory infections and their morbidity and mortality are markedly reduced with influenza vaccination. To define the effects of influenza and the benefits of influenza vaccination in elderly people with chronic lung disease, Nichol et al conducted a retrospective, multiseason cohort study in a large managed-care organization. The outcomes in vaccinated and unvaccinated individuals were compared after adjustment for baseline demographics and health characteristics. This study showed that vaccination rates were >70%. Hospitalization rates for patients not vaccinated for pneumonia and influenza were twice as high in the influenza season as they were in the interim (noninfluenza) periods (Figure 8-13). Vaccinated patients had fewer outpatient visits, fewer hospitalizations, and fewer deaths. Consequently, the influenza vaccine should be given to patients with COPD.

The polyvalent vaccine, based on pneumococcal capsule serotypes, has been shown to be effective in preventing pneumococcal bacteremia and pneumonia. The available 23 serotype vaccine has been shown to have an aggregate efficacy of more than 60%. The efficacy tends to decline with age and patient's immune state. The vaccine is also recommended for patients with COPD. There are no contraindications for use of either the pneumococcal or the influenza vaccine immediately after an episode of pneumonia or acute exacerbation of COPD. Vaccines can be given simultaneously without affecting their potency. There are no other vaccines available for adults to prevent lower respiratory tract infections. Vaccines intended to prevent infections from atypical *Haemophilus* sp or *Pseudomonas* sp are being developed but are not yet available.

Suggested Readings

Adams SG, Anzueto A: Antibiotic therapy in acute exacerbations of chronic bronchitis. *Semin Respir Infect* 2000;15:234-247.

Albert RK, Martin TR, Lewis SW: Controlled clinical trial of methylprednisolone in patients with chronic bronchitis and acute respiratory insufficiency. *Ann Intern Med* 1980;92:753-758.

Anzueto A, Rizzo JA, Grossman RF: The infection-free interval: its use in evaluating antimicrobial treatment of acute exacerbation of chronic bronchitis. *Clin Infect Dis* 1999;28:1344-1345.

Au DH, Lemaitre RN, Curtis JR, et al: The risk of myocardial infarction associated with inhaled beta-adrenoceptor agonists. *Am J Respir Crit Care Med* 2000;161(3 pt 1):827-830.

Ball P, Harris JM, Lowson D, et al: Acute infective exacerbations of chronic bronchitis. *QJM* 1995;88:61-68.

Berry RB, Shinto RA, Wong FH, et al: Nebulizer vs spacer for bronchodilator delivery in patients hospitalized for acute exacerbations of COPD. *Chest* 1989;96:1241-1246.

Celli BR, MacNee W, ATS/ERS Task Force: Standards for the diagnosis and treatment of patients with COPD: a summary of the ATS/ERS position paper. *Eur Respir J* 2004;23:932-946.

Connors AF Jr, Dawson NV, Thomas C, et al: Outcomes following acute exacerbation of severe chronic obstructive lung disease. The SUPPORT investigators (Study to Understand Prognoses and Preferences for Outcomes and Risks of Treatments). *Am J Respir Crit Care Med* 1996;154(4 pt 1):959-967.

Cook D, Guyatt G, Wong E, et al: Regular versus as-needed short-acting inhaled beta-agonist therapy for chronic obstructive pulmonary disease. *Am J Respir Crit Care Med* 2001;163:85-90.

Davies L, Angus RM, Calverley PM: Oral corticosteroids in patients admitted to hospital with exacerbations of chronic obstructive pulmonary disease: a prospective randomised controlled trial. *Lancet* 1999;354:456-460.

Dhand R, Jubran A, Tobin MJ: Bronchodilator delivery by metered-dose inhaler in ventilator-supported patients. *Am J Respir Crit Care Med* 1995;151:1827-1833.

Duarte AG, Dhand R, Reid R, et al: Serum albuterol levels in mechanically ventilated patients and healthy subjects after metered-dose inhaler administration. *Am J Respir Crit Care Med* 1996;154(6 pt 1): 1658-1663.

Eller J, Ede A, Schaberg T, et al: Infective exacerbations of chronic bronchitis: relation between bacteriologic etiology and lung function. *Chest* 1998;113:1542-1548.

Emerman CL, Cydulka RK: Evaluation of high-yield criteria for chest radiography in acute exacerbation of chronic obstructive pulmonary disease. *Ann Emerg Med* 1993;22:680-684.

Emerman CL, Effron D, Lukens TW: Spirometric criteria for hospital admission of patients with acute exacerbations of COPD. *Chest* 1991;99:595-599.

Global Strategy for Diagnosis, Management, and Prevention of COPD. 2006 Update.

Gompertz S, O'Brien C, Bayley DL, et al: Changes in bronchial inflammation during acute exacerbations of chronic bronchitis. *Eur Respir J* 2001;17:1112-1119.

Hudson LD, Monti CM: Rationale and use of corticosteroids in chronic obstructive pulmonary disease. *Med Clin North Am* 1990;74:661-690.

Karpel JP, Pesin J, Greenberg D, et al: A comparison of the effects of ipratropium bromide and metaproterenol sulfate in acute exacerbations of COPD. *Chest* 1990;98:835-839.

Madison JM, Irwin RS: Chronic obstructive pulmonary disease. *Lancet* 1998;352:467-473.

Maltais F, Ostinelli J, Bourbeau J, et al: Comparison of nebulized budesonide and oral prednisolone with placebo in the treatment of acute exacerbations of chronic obstructive pulmonary disease: a randomized controlled trial. *Am J Respir Crit Care Med* 2002;165: 698-703.

Miravitlles M, Espinosa C, Fernandez-Laso E, et al: Relationship between bacterial flora in sputum and functional impairment in patients with acute exacerbations of COPD. Study Group of Bacterial Infection in COPD. *Chest* 1999;116:40-46.

Moayyedi P, Congleton J, Page RL, et al: Comparison of nebulised salbutamol and ipratropium bromide with salbutamol alone in the treatment of chronic obstructive pulmonary disease. *Thorax* 1995;50:834-837.

Monso E, Ruiz J, Rosell A, et al: Bacterial infection in chronic obstructive pulmonary disease. A study of stable and exacerbated outpatients using the protected specimen brush. *Am J Respir Crit Care Med* 1995;152(4 pt 1):1316-1320.

Murphy TF, Sethi S: Bacterial infection in chronic obstructive pulmonary disease. *Am Rev Respir Dis* 1992;146:1067-1083.

Murray CJ, Lopez AD: Alternative projections of mortality and disability by cause 1990-2020: Global Burden of Disease Study. *Lancet* 1997;349:1498-1504.

Niederman MS, Mandell LA, Anzueto A, et al: Guidelines for the management of adults with community-acquired pneumonia. Diagnosis, assessment of severity, antimicrobial therapy, and prevention. *Am J Respir Crit Care Med* 2001;163:1730-1754.

Niewoehner DE, Erbland ML, Deupree RH, et al: Effect of systemic glucocorticoids on exacerbations of chronic obstructive pulmonary disease. Department of Veterans Affairs Cooperative Study Group. *N Engl J Med* 1999;340:1941-1947.

Nouira S, Marghli S, Belghith M, et al: Once daily oral ofloxacin in chronic obstructive pulmonary disease exacerbation requiring mechanical ventilation: a randomised placebo-controlled trial. *Lancet* 2001;358:2020-2025.

O'Driscoll BR, Taylor RJ, Horsley MG, et al: Nebulised salbutamol with and without ipratropium bromide in acute airflow obstruction. *Lancet* 1989;1:1418-1420.

Pallares R, Linares J, Vadillo M, et al: Resistance to penicillin and cephalosporin and mortality from severe pneumococcal pneumonia in Barcelona, Spain. *N Engl J Med* 1995;333:474-480.

Peters KD, Kochanek KD, Murphy SL: Deaths: final data for 1996. *Natl Vital Stat Rep* 1998;47:1-100.

Rice KL, Leatherman JW, Duane PG, et al: Aminophylline for acute exacerbations of chronic obstructive pulmonary disease. A controlled trial. *Ann Intern Med* 1987;107:305-309.

Seemungal T, Harper-Owen R, Bhowmik A, et al: Respiratory viruses, symptoms, and inflammatory markers in acute exacerbations and stable chronic obstructive pulmonary disease. *Am J Respir Crit Care Med* 2001;164:1618-1623.

Seidenfeld JJ, Jones WN, Moss RE, et al: Intravenous aminophylline in the treatment of acute bronchospastic exacerbations of chronic obstructive pulmonary disease. *Ann Emerg Med* 1984;13:248-252.

Seneff MG, Wagner DP, Wagner RP, et al: Hospital and 1-year survival of patients admitted to intensive care units with acute exacerbation of chronic obstructive pulmonary disease. *JAMA* 1995;274:1852-1857.

Sethi S, Muscarella K, Evans N, et al: Airway inflammation and etiology of acute exacerbations of chronic bronchitis. *Chest* 2000;118:1557-1565.

Sethi S, Evans N, Grant BJ, et al: New strains of bacteria and exacerbations of chronic obstructive pulmonary disease. *New Engl J Med* 2002;347:465-471.

Shrestha M, O'Brien T, Haddox R, et al: Decreased duration of emergency department treatment of chronic obstructive pulmonary disease exacerbations with the addition of ipratropium bromide to beta-agonist therapy. *Ann Emerg Med* 1991;20:1206-1209.

Smith CB, Golden CA, Kanner RE, et al: Haemophilus influenzae and Haemophilus parainfluenzae in chronic obstructive pulmonary disease. *Lancet* 1976;1:1253-1255.

Statistical Abstract of the United States 1997. Available at: http://www.census.gov. Accessed November 9, 2006.

Thompson WH, Nielson CP, Carvalho P, et al: Controlled trial of oral prednisone in outpatients with acute COPD exacerbation. *Am J Respir Crit Care Med* 1996;154:407-412.

Thornsberry C, Ogilvie P, Kahn J, et al: Surveillance of antimicrobial resistance in Streptococcus pneumoniae, Haemophilus influenzae, and Moraxella catarrhalis in the United States in 1996-1997 respiratory season. The Laboratory Investigator Group. *Diag Microbiol Infect Dis* 1997;29:249-257.

Tsai TW, Gallagher EJ, Lombardi G, et al: Guidelines for the selective ordering of admission chest radiography in adult obstructive airway disease. *Ann Emerg Med* 1993;22:1854-1858.

Turner MO, Patel A, Ginsburg S, et al: Bronchodilator delivery in acute airflow obstruction. A meta-analysis. *Arch Intern Med* 1997;157:1736-1744.

Wilson R, Schentag JJ, Ball P, et al: A comparison of gemifloxacin and clarithromycin in acute exacerbations of chronic bronchitis and long-term clinical outcomes. *Clin Ther* 2002;24:639-652.

Chapter 9

Quality of Life and Ethical Considerations

The treatment of chronic obstructive pulmonary disease (COPD) is largely directed toward relief of symptoms. More recently, there has been an emphasis on addressing the patient's functional status and the overall economic impact of the disease. In addition to physical limitations, patients with COPD commonly experience anxiety and/or depression, as well as a diminished quality of life (QOL). Furthermore, several studies demonstrated that current and intermittent smokers had worse mental health as evidenced by lower mental component scale (MCS) scores on the 36-item, short-form health survey (SF-36), and more frequent diagnoses of depression, posttraumatic stress disorder (PTSD), and schizophrenia than former smokers. In addition, current smokers have worse mental health than intermittent smokers. Investigators examined the relationship between smoking status and health-related quality of life in the general population and have demonstrated that active cigarette smoking relates to poor quality of life. Some studies have reported an initial increase in anxiety and depression within the first 6 months following smoking cessation. However, other studies have demonstrated that former smokers experience better perceived mental and physical health than current smokers, especially after the initial period of smoking cessation.

Health status and QOL have been recognized as important outcomes in medical care. The impact of a disease on an individual's ability to carry out daily activities and derive personal fulfillment in life may determine that person's health status. Quality of life is considered a key component of health status and also includes environmental aspects affected by health and treatment. COPD guidelines from the Global Initiative for Chronic Obstructive Lung Disease (GOLD) and the ATS/ERS consensus statement recognize that pharmacologic treatment not only has an impact on pulmonary function but can also improve overall health status.

Instruments Available to Measure QOL
Generic Questionnaires
These questionnaires were developed to assess a broad range of diseases and disease components. They are used to make valuable comparisons between various health conditions and establish an overall assessment of the total impact of the disease and treatment regimen on a patient's life. The generic questionnaires are often insensitive in mild-to-moderate conditions and in detecting minor physiologic changes in clinical status.

Short-Form 36-item (SF-36) Questionnaire
This is a widely used questionnaire and is considered advantageous because of its brief layout and translation into several different languages. This instrument assesses eight domains and identifies limitations in physical activity, social activity, daily roles, bodily pain, general mental health, vitality, and general health problems. The questionnaire uses variable scaling depending on each question (eg, very good/good/poor or mild/moderate/severe).

Sickness Impact Profile (SIP)
This questionnaire was designed to measure the effect of a disease on a patient's physical and emotional functioning on the day the test is administered. The instrument consists of 136 questions, which may be categorized into

sleep and rest, eating, work, home management, recreation and pastimes, ambulation, mobility, body care and movement, social interaction, alertness, emotional behavior, and communication. Each category is included in one of two domains, psychosocial or physical. The overall scores, domain scores, and category scores are calculated. This questionnaire has the disadvantage of a long administration time.

Inventory of Subjective Health (ISH)

This questionnaire consists of 21 questions relating to subjective physical complaints, such as tiredness, chest and heart problems, gastric problems, indigestion, and headache. Most complaints are grouped according to the anatomy affected, while the remaining complaints are classified as overall physical health. The overall ISH score reflects the number of physical complaints with higher scores representing a greater number of complaints.

Nottingham Health Profile (NHP)

This is a self-administered questionnaire designed to assess perceived physical, emotional, and social health dysfunctions, with emphasis on the patient's subjective perception. Questions were taken from the SIP and interviews with patients who have acute or chronic diseases. The instrument consists of 38 questions, categorized into 6 dimensions, including physical mobility (8 questions), pain (8 questions), social isolation (5 questions), emotional reactions (9 questions), energy (3 questions), and sleep (5 questions). Mean overall scores and scores for each dimension are calculated, and range from 0 to 100, with higher scores representing greater health complaints.

COPD Disease-specific Questionnaires

These instruments were designed to determine the key components that impact a specific disease or health condition. The main advantage is that they may detect small physiologic changes more easily than a generic questionnaire and provide more detail on which clinical variables are most affected by treatment.

Chronic Respiratory Disease Questionnaire (CRDQ)

This was the first instrument designed to measure QOL in COPD. The questionnaire can either be given orally by an interviewer or self administered. The instrument has 20 questions separated into four domains: dyspnea, fatigue, emotional functioning, and mastery. For the dyspnea domain, the patient chooses five activities that cause the greatest amount of dyspnea, thereby 'individualizing' the questionnaire. Scores range from 1-7, with 1 indicating total impairment and 7 indicating no impairment. Results are expressed as a mean score for each domain and a mean overall score. A minimum change of 0.5 indicates a clinically important change. This instrument emphasizes the emotional impact of COPD: frustrations, restlessness, embarrassment, worries, and depression.

St. George's Respiratory Questionnaire (SGRQ)

This is one of the most widely used instruments to assess QOL in patients with asthma or COPD. This questionnaire was designed to quantify the impact of chronic airflow limitation on health and well-being. The instrument addresses the impact of respiratory conditions on an individual's social life, household activities, and employment, and is sufficiently sensitive to respond to changes in disease activity. The questionnaire consists of 50 questions, with two to five responses for each question. Responses are expressed as an overall score and three subscores for symptoms, activities, and impact. These components measure *Symptoms* (distress caused by respiratory symptoms), *Activity* (effects of disturbances to mobility and physical activity), and *Impacts* (quantifying the psychosocial impact of disease). A number of items in the symptoms components relate to the frequency of symptoms over the previous year. Both the activity and impacts components relate to the patient's current state. Results are expressed as a percentile, with 0% representing the best possible score and 100% representing the worst. A minimum change of 4% or 4 units (U) for each domain and the total score indicates a clinically important response to treatment.

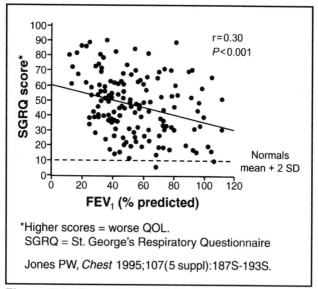

Figure 9-1: Correlation of QOL Scores (SGRQ) with FEV_1 in COPD patients.

Relationship Between Spirometry and Quality of Life

Spirometry has been the main objective parameter used to evaluate patients with COPD. There is controversy related to the relationship between spirometry and changes in a patient's QOL. Figure 9-1 shows a scattergram from a study by Jones et al that reflects the regression plot between the SGRQ and postbronchodilator forced expiratory volume in 1 second (FEV_1) (as percentage predicted) in patients with COPD. This study was performed in patients with a range of disease severity who were receiving treatment at the time of the study. A high questionnaire score (maximum 100) indicates worse QOL. The data presented illustrate that only a weak correlation exists between loss of FEV_1 and impaired QOL.

A considerable proportion of patients had relatively mild disease, with spirometric values on the day of testing that lay within the normal range. The authors observed that even in these patients, the SGRQ scores were well above those for an age-matched normal population, suggesting that spirometry may be relatively insensitive in detecting early effects of COPD on patients.

QOL Outcomes for Patients Receiving Pharmacologic and Pulmonary Rehabilitation Treatment for COPD

Patient-reported health outcomes may result in more comprehensive COPD management. Clinical studies have demonstrated the impact of pharmacologic treatment on QOL and health status in COPD. Chronic obstructive pulmonary disease guidelines support regular treatment with long-active bronchodilators including long-acting β-agonists (LABAs) and tiotropium (Spiriva®) to improve health status, and recommend them over short-acting bronchodilators for sustained improvements in QOL.

Results from a 6-week clinical study showed formoterol (Foradil®) treatment (12 μg b.i.d.) significantly improved the activities domain of the SGRQ (P=0.041) as well as the total SGRQ score (P=0.0410) compared with placebo (Figure 9-2). Significant improvements in the role-emotional and social functioning domains of the SF-36 were observed with formoterol treatment compared with placebo treatment (P=0.0327).These effects have also been reported with salmeterol (Serevent Diskus®) (Figure 9-3). After a 16-week, dose-ranging study comparing salmeterol (50 μg and 100 μg b.i.d.) with placebo treatment, treatment with salmeterol (50 μg b.i.d.) resulted in clinically significant improvements (>4 U) in the total SGRQ score and the impact domain score compared with placebo. However, treatment with salmeterol 100 μg b.i.d. was comparable to placebo, likely caused by the increased side effects (eg, tremor). Furthermore, although salmeterol 50 μg b.i.d. significantly improved QOL, only a

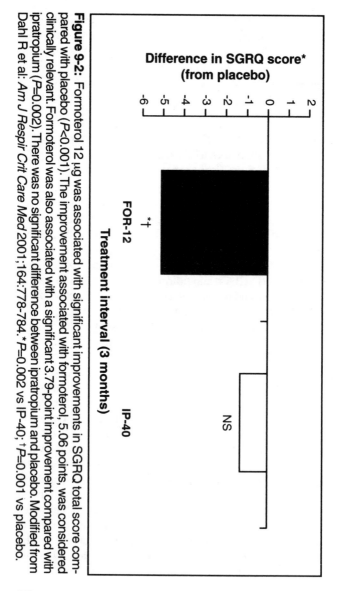

Figure 9-2: Formoterol 12 µg was associated with significant improvements in SGRQ total score compared with placebo (*P*<0.001). The improvement associated with formoterol, 5.06 points, was considered clinically relevant. Formoterol was also associated with a significant 3.79-point improvement compared with ipratropium (*P*=0.002). There was no significant difference between ipratropium and placebo. Modified from Dahl R et al: *Am J Respir Crit Care Med* 2001;164:778-784. *P*=0.002 vs IP-40; †*P*=0.001 vs placebo.

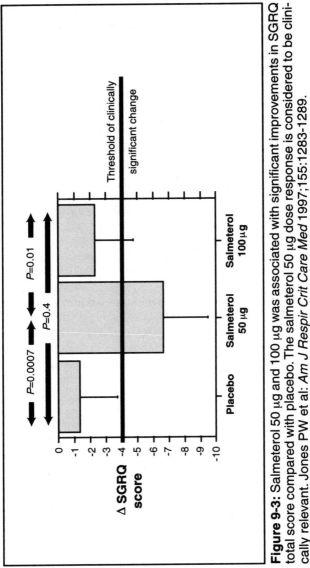

Figure 9-3: Salmeterol 50 μg and 100 μg was associated with significant improvements in SGRQ total score compared with placebo. The salmeterol 50 μg dose response is considered to be clinically relevant. Jones PW et al: *Am J Respir Crit Care Med* 1997;155:1283-1289.

modest change in FEV_1 occurred, demonstrating a weak correlation between clinical status and QOL.

Studies using long-active anticholinergics have shown significant improvements in patients' QOL. Following 1 year of treatment with tiotropium (18 μg) or placebo, QOL was assessed using both the SGRQ (Figure 9-4 and Figure 9-5) and the SF-36 (Figure 9-6 A, B). Compared with placebo, tiotropium significantly improved the total SGRQ score and each SGRQ domain ($P<0.05$), as well as the vitality and social function domains of the SF-36 ($P<0.05$). Tiotropium was significantly more effective than placebo in improving physical health-related scores (except bodily pain). For the mental health domains, tiotropium was more effective than placebo in vitality and social function domains at day 344. The two treatment groups were similar for other mental health domains. In a 6-month comparative study, tiotropium treatment (18 μg q.d.) significantly improved total and impact SGRQ scores (5.14 U and 5.24 U, respectively; $P<0.05$) compared with placebo, whereas salmeterol treatment (50 μg b.i.d.) did not result in any clinically significant improvements in the total SGRQ score (3.54 U, $P=0.39$) and impact domain (2.37 U; $P=0.98$) compared with placebo treatment. Following 1 year of treatment, tiotropium (18 μg q.d.) produced superior improvements in the total SGRQ score compared with ipratropium (40 μg q.i.d.; $P<0.05$). Tiotropium treatment also resulted in significantly greater improvements in the SGRQ impact domain score ($P=0.004$), and more patients receiving tiotropium treatment achieved a clinically meaningful response (>4 U) compared with patients receiving ipratropium treatment (52% vs 35%; $P=0.001$).

GOLD guidelines recommend ICS therapy only in patients with severe-to-very-severe COPD and during acute exacerbations. ICS treatment reduces the rate of exacerbations, thereby improving health status. Results from a 3-year study showed that a high dose of fluticasone propionate (Advair Diskus®, Flonase®, Flovent® HFA) (500 μg b.i.d.) significantly reduced the rate of deterioration of the total SGRQ

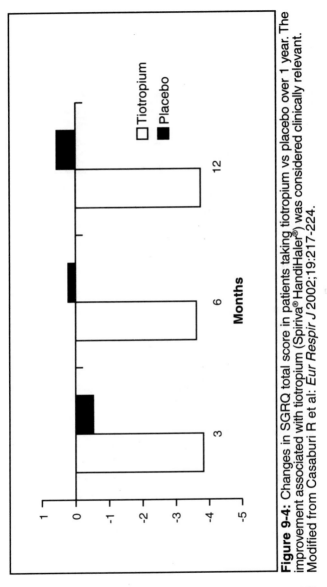

Figure 9-4: Changes in SGRQ total score in patients taking tiotropium vs placebo over 1 year. The improvement associated with tiotropium (Spiriva®HandiHaler®) was considered clinically relevant. Modified from Casaburi R et al: *Eur Respir J* 2002;19:217-224.

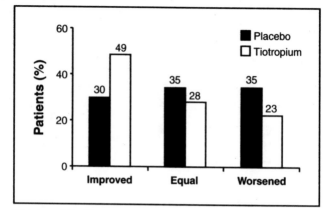

Figure 9-5: Percentage of patients with 4-unit change in SGRQ total score, tiotropium vs placebo, based on overall patient response. Modified from Casaburi R et al: *Eur Respir J* 2002;19:217-224.

score compared with placebo treatment ($P<0.004$). Significant improvements were also observed in the SF-36 domains in physical function ($P<0.005$), energy/vitality ($P<0.02$), physical role limitation ($P<0.05$), and mental health ($P<0.005$).

Fixed combination therapies of an ICS and LABA have also shown a significant improvement in patient QOL. In a 12-month study, patients were randomized to treatment with budesonide/formoterol (320 μg b.i.d./9 μg b.i.d.), budesonide (400 μg b.i.d.), formoterol (9 μg b.i.d.), or placebo. Although all active treatment groups demonstrated improved total SGRQ scores compared with placebo, combination therapy with budesonide/formoterol resulted in the greatest improvement. Budesonide/formoterol combination treatment also resulted in significant improvements compared with budesonide and formoterol treatment given alone for the activity ($P<0.05$) and impact domain scores of the SGRQ ($P<0.001$ vs budesonide and $P<0.05$ vs formoterol). Similar results are reported following 12

6A

Treatment Differences at Day 344

Domain	Difference	P
Physical function	4.6	≤ 0.001
Role physical	9.0	≤ 0.001
Pain	2.5	ns
General physical health	4.0	≤ 0.001
Physical health summary	2.4	≤ 0.001

6B

Treatment Differences at Day 344

Domain	Difference	P
Vitality	3.2	≤ 0.01
Social function	3.9	0.01
Role emotional	4.0	ns
General mental health	0.8	ns
Mental health summary	0.6	ns

Figure 9-6: SF-36 Physical Health Domains (6A) and Mental Health Domains (6B) in patients treated with tiotropium or placebo for 1 year. Modified from Casaburi R et al: *Eur Resp J* 2002;19:217-224.

months of treatment with fluticasone propionate/salmeterol (500/50 µg b.i.d.), fluticasone, salmeterol, or placebo, but only the combination treatment resulted in significant improvements in SGRQ scores compared with placebo and fluticasone alone ($P < 0.01$) (Figure 9-7).

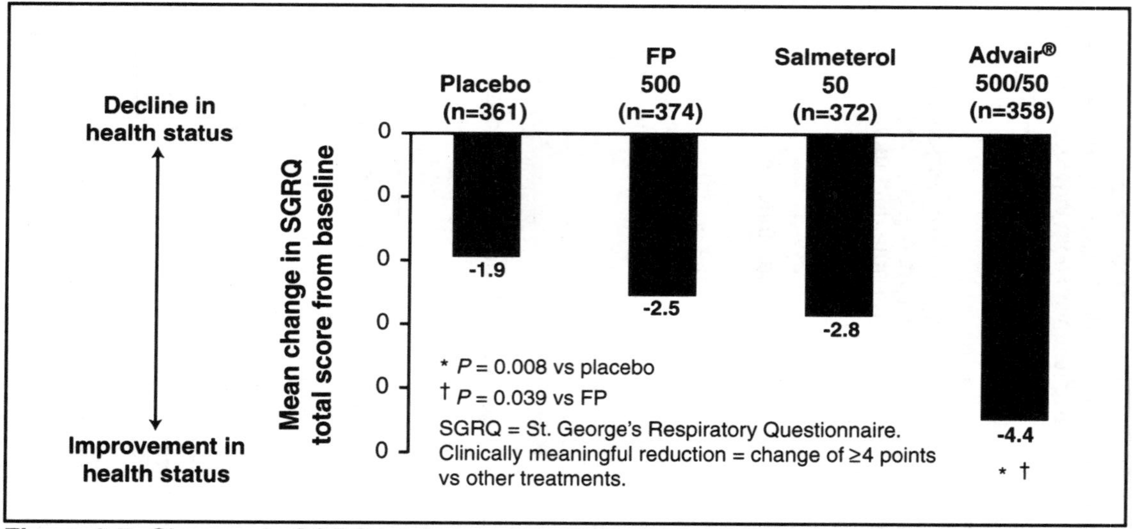

Figure 9-7: Changes in SGRQ total score in patients taking fluticasone, salmeterol, fixed combination of fluticasone/salmeterol vs placebo. The improvement associated with fixed combination of fluticasone/salmeterol was considered clinically relevant. Jones PW et al: Presented at American Thoracic Society meeting, May 17-22, 2002, Atlanta, GA.

184

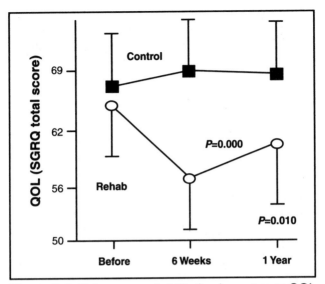

Figure 9-8: Pulmonary rehabilitation impact over QOL based on SGRQ response at 1 year. There is a significant improvement in patients treated who completed a pulmonary rehabilitation program. Adapted from Griffiths TL et al: *Lancet* 2000;355:362-368.

A controlled trial (N=200) assessing the effects of pulmonary rehabilitation in patients with COPD showed short- and long-term effects in outpatients at a multidisciplinary pulmonary rehabilitation unit (Figure 9-8). Exercise and QOL reports were better in the rehabilitation group compared with the control group. Small declines over 1 year were found for both exercise capacity and QOL for the control group, and positive differences for the rehabilitation group, although in some cases small, were deemed significant.

Conclusion

Improving QOL in patients with COPD is an essential component of a successful management approach. COPD guidelines recommend pharmacologic therapy to improve overall health status. Regular treatment with a long-active bronchodilator, alone or in combination, has been shown to improve patients' health status.

Ethical Considerations

The clinical profile of a COPD patient in the last years of life involves several conditions besides the patient's lung function. A summary of this profile is summarized in Table 9-1. Thus, caregivers must recognize and address the ethical dilemmas that arise in caring for patients with advanced COPD, assist patients with advance care planning, and understand the perspectives of patients with advanced lung disease who may face end-of-life decisions. Patients with moderate-to-severe COPD experience frequent acute exacerbations, each of which can result in an acute respiratory failure and a possible need for ventilatory support. These exacerbations can result in significant morbidity and even mortality. Patients with COPD exacerbations and hypercapnia that require invasive mechanical ventilation, have hospital discharge survival rates as low as 76%. Also, only 59% of patients are still alive 1 year later. Furthermore, the patient's QOL after discharge is frequently poor because of persistent respiratory symptoms. This guarded prognosis presents significant ethical dilemmas for both the patient and the caregiver.

Patients with COPD will benefit from advance care planning. Advance care planning is derived from the principle of patient autonomy, wherein a patient directs his or her own health-care decisions. Unfortunately, most patients with advanced COPD have not discussed their end-of-life wishes with their physicians or other caregivers. Formal written documents, such as living wills and durable powers of healthcare, have not fulfilled their goals to improve end-of-life care. Comprehensive advance care planning depends on care tailored to a patient's individual needs to fulfill his or her psychological, emotional, and spiritual needs.

The emphasis of discussions on end-of-life care may shift from patient-physician discussions on the use of life-supportive interventions to patient-family-friend communication. This communication strengthens relationships and shares decisions regarding life-supportive care. Physicians, with their patients' permission, can promote a dialogue for advance-care planning by involving families and encouraging discussions within families regarding the end-of-life decisions that patients may eventually face. Caregivers can enrich these discussions by providing patients with educational materials and resources that enhance informed decisions.

Hospice care could be a consideration for patients with severe COPD. Hospices are organized programs of support services for patients in the advanced stages of a terminal illness (with their families). Although hospices serve dying patients regardless of diagnosis, limited available evidence suggests that these programs are relatively underused by patients dying of nonmalignant lung diseases. The unpredictability of death from advanced lung disease may be a likely reason for the underuse of these services in patients with COPD. Certain limitations on federal and private insurance coverage for patients with advanced lung disease probably contribute as well. For hospice benefits, Medicare requires indication from the physician that the patient is terminally ill and has fewer than 6 months to live. Hospice care seeks neither to prolong life nor to hasten death. Its purpose is to maximize comfort, dignity, and the QOL for the dying and to help bereaved survivors cope with their loss. For those patients who do enroll, hospice offers expert palliation of physical, psychological, social, and spiritual distress, as well as practical support for home-care needs, hospitalization for short-term control of symptoms, and inpatient respite care for relief of home caregivers. Hospice workers view dying as an active phase of life filled with the pursuit of goals that patients and family members wish to complete before or shortly after the end of life.

Suggested Readings

Casaburi R, Mahler DA, Jones PW, et al: A long-term evaluation of once-daily inhaled tiotropium in chronic obstructive pulmonary disease. *Eur Respir J* 2002;19:217-224.

Celli BR, MacNee W, ATS/ERS Task Force: Standards for the diagnosis and treatment of patients with COPD: a summary of the ATS/ERS position paper. *Eur Respir J* 2004;23:932-946.

Dahl R, Greefhorst LA, Nowak D, et al: Inhaled formoterol dry powder versus ipratropium bromide in chronic obstructive pulmonary disease. *Am J Respir Crit Care Med* 2001;164:778-784.

Fabbri L, Pauwels RA, Hurd S: Global Strategy for the Diagnosis, Management, and Prevention of Chronic Obstructive Pulmonary Disease: GOLD Executive Summary updated 2003. *COPD* 2004;1:105-141; discussion 103-104.

Global Strategy for Diagnosis, Management, and Prevention of COPD. 2006 Update.

Guyatt GH, Berman LB, et al: A measure of quality of life for clinical trials in chronic lung disease. *Thorax* 1987;42:773-778.

Jones PW: Issues concerning health-related quality of life in COPD. *Chest* 1995;107(5 suppl):187S-193S.

Jones PW, Quirk FH, et al: A self-complete measure of health status in chronic airflow limitation. The St. George's Respiratory Questionnaire. *Am Rev Respir Dis* 1992;145:1321-1327.

Katz S, Ford AB, Moskowitz RW, et al: Studies of illness in the aged. The index of ADL: a standardized measure of biological and psychosocial function. *JAMA* 1963;185:914-919.

Vincken W, van Noord JA, Greefhorst AP, et al: Improved health outcomes in patients with COPD during 1 yr treatment with tiotropium. *Eur Respir J* 2002;19:209-216.

Ware JE, ed. *The SF-36 Health Survey Manual Interpretation Guide.* Boston, MA, Nimrod Press, 1993.

Ware JE Jr, Gandek B: Overview of the SF-36 Health Survey and the International Quality of Life Assessment (IQOLA) Project. *J Clin Epidemiol* 1998;51:903-912.

Index